KETO DIET
for Women Over 50

The Ultimate Ketogenic Diet Guide For Senior to Lose Weight & Balance Hormones with 100 Healthy, Delicious, Low-Carb Recipes and an In____ Good 28-days Meal P___

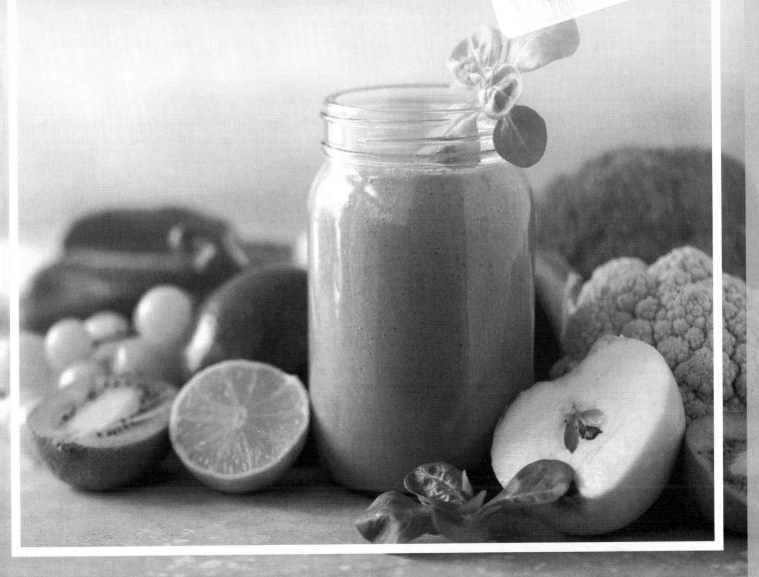

TABLE OF CONTENTS

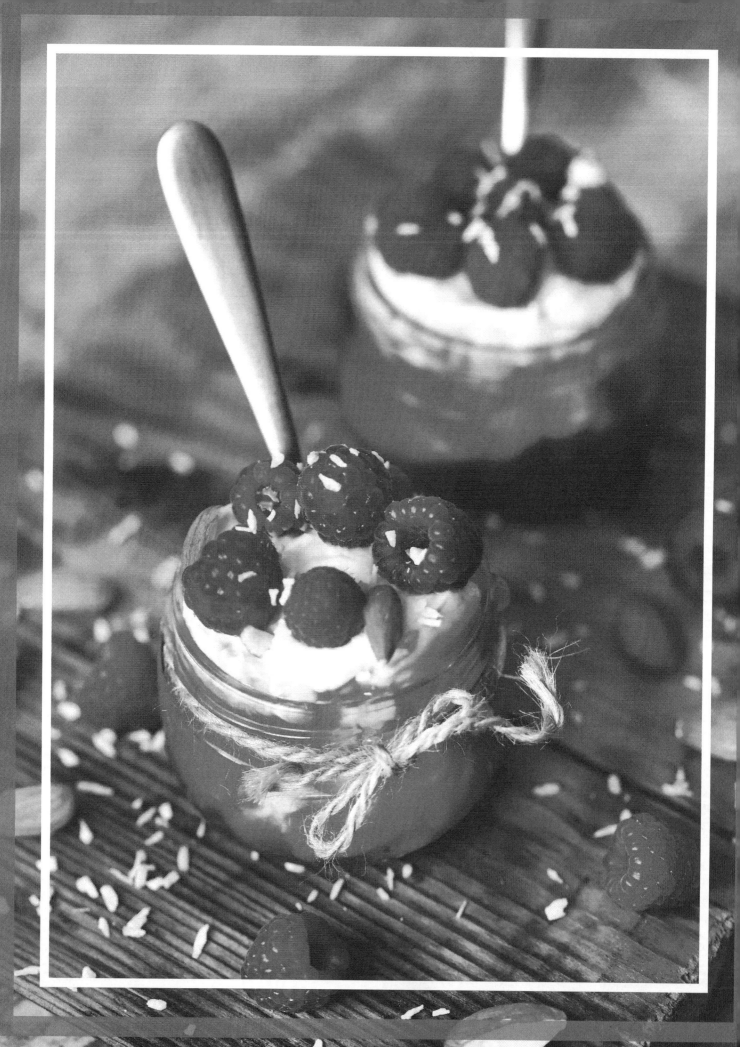

INTRODUCTION

As we age, we naturally look for ways to hold onto our youth and energy. It's not uncommon to think about things that promote anti-aging. Products and lifestyle changes are advertised everywhere, and they are designed to catch your attention, as you grapple with the reality of what it means to be a 50+-year-old woman in our society. Even if you aren't eating for the purposes of anti-aging yet, you have likely thought about it in terms of the way you treat your skin and hair, for example. The great thing about the Keto diet is that it supports maximum health from the inside out; working hard to make sure that you are in the best shape that you can be in.

The ketogenic diet has many important aspects and information that you need to know as someone who wants to try this diet. It is important to remember the warning that we have given you at the beginning of the book that this is not a diet that is safe and that doctors recommend you don't try it; or if you are going to attempt it, remember that you shouldn't do so for longer than six months and even then never without the constant supervision of a doctor or, at the very least, a doctor knowing that you're doing this and you are following their guidelines and words exactly so that they can make sure that you are safe.

Your body burns sugars, which are found in carbohydrates, and fats throughout the day to give you energy. When you reduce your intake of carbohydrates, your body is no longer able to use these sugars as an energy source and switches to burning fat instead. This process is called ketosis, and it forms the foundation of the keto diet.

The keto diet will result in increased brain function and the ability to focus. The brain typically uses sugar to fuel its processes, but the consumption of sugar has its problems. The mind can easily switch to using ketones for fuel and energy. Remember that ketones are the by-product of

Ketosis that makes you burn fat. The keto diet was used by doctors to control seizures in patients long before medications were invented.

As many people are using this diet to their benefit, knowing your food is one of the biggest parts of this, and it becomes easier once you begin to use this in your daily life. One of the best things you can do is pay attention to the food that your eating and how it affects your body and mind. You will notice that this diet can make you sick, which isn't a good thing and it's one of the things the doctors warn against. For this reason, it's very important to pay attention to what you're eating and how you're feeling at the same time. Another warning that we have said you need to pay attention to is that you will need to make sure that your ketogenic 'flu' isn't the result of something more serious. As people are being told that this is normal, this book has brought you the knowledge you need to be able to know why it's not.

When the keto diet helps you lose weight, it also reduces your risk of cardiovascular disease. When you lose weight and decrease the amount of fat and cholesterol in the body, there will be less to accumulate in the arteries, and the blood will naturally flow better with less restriction.

Adopting the keto way of life will also help eliminate problems with the kidneys and improve their function. Kidney stones and gout are caused mainly by the elevation of certain urine chemicals that help create uric acid, which we eliminate in the bathroom. When ketones begin to rise, the acid in urine will briefly increase as your body begins to eliminate all of the waste products from the metabolized fats. However, the level will decrease and remain lower than before as long as you are on the keto diet.

You will find plenty of delicious recipes in this book that will get you started on your new journey. The weekly meal plans are suggestions you can follow, and feel free to mix the meals up to suit your needs. This plan is a four-week plan to get you started.

CHAPTER 1

What is Keto Diet and Ketosis

WHAT IS KETO DIET

The keto diet was developed in 1924 by Dr. Russel as a treatment of epileptic patients. However, over time, there are beneficial aspects of this diet that people are applying in their lives and enhancing their livelihood. He observed that when the body is in ketosis, it will prevent the onset of epileptic symptoms, hence curing the condition. There are other benefits of the diet, which include: healing of brain injuries, preventing heart attack, maintaining a perfect level of blood glucose, treating autism, among others.

Since the diet lacks carbohydrates, the ketogenic diet is rich in fats and proteins. It includes meals with plenty of eggs, meats, cheeses, fish, butter, oils, and seeds, as well as fibrous vegetables. The body likes to utilize glucose for energy; however, this is not the most efficient source of energy because it brings serious health problems such as obesity, diabetes, among other problems associated with a high carbohydrate diet. Glucose is the primary source of energy for your cells in the body, and when the levels of glucose are high, they are not burnt; and this, in turn, will result in the conversion of the glucose molecules to glycogen. Glycogen is stored in the peripheral and visceral organs leading to obesity.

However, as we age, we need foods that will give us adequate energy and are easily metabolized to reduce the chances of developing lifestyle diseases such as diabetes. The keto diet brings the body to ketosis; the body will utilize the fats for energy. The reason for writing this book is for people over 50 years to make the right choice when it comes to diet. The book will help you understand various diets that will suit your age and rejuvenate your cells while preventing any kind of illnesses.

When you follow the ketogenic diet, you will be able to avoid cravings, such as those of sugar, and choose something healthier and one which will promote cell development. You will feel fitter, healthier, and sharper.

Naturally, counting calories and ingesting less of them will help you lose weight, but if not, be careful, as you might not eat the right calories and may end up losing muscle mass. Counting macros instead can counter this. 100 calories of avocado (fat) are better than 100 calories of a doughnut (carb). With the Keto diet, it's important to be aware of your carbs-to-protein and fat ratio. Normally, to maintain ketosis, most people aim for 50 grams or fewer carbs a day.

When calculating macros, you just add up the grams of fat, carbs, and protein you ate that day. Let's say you had 10 saltine crackers, and a serving size is 5 crackers. You would then multiply the numbers on the label by 28g of fat, 20g of carbs, and 2g of protein. Document this process, and you can visually see where your number runs high in carbs.

There are several ways you can document your process, and you're encouraged to try all that works for you. You really will have to be diligent in this diet to ensure you're eating the proper proportion of macronutrients, and it may become endlessly helpful for you to keep track of your process — not to mention your day-to-day consumption.

You might consider just keeping tabs on your progress with a series of notes on your phone, but it's possible that you need a little more time to devote some careful attention to this procedure. In that case, you might try journaling about your intake, your process, and its outcomes. You may also feel drawn to using an app that could help you keep track of these same things. Finally, you could try using a dry erase board to keep tabs on your meal plan or menu for the week. More creative readers will extrapolate far more options beyond just these few provided.

No matter what you do, you're encouraged — at least for the first few weeks of your diet — to be conscientious of your food labels and keep track of what you're eating in a journal or an app. It's also good to have a scale for your household and a travel scale for the on-the-go. It's such that not all keto-friendly products have nutrition labels on them. It might be up to you to determine how much of what you're eating.

The keto diet is a very healthy and natural way to lose weight, but as with most new health regimens, there can be a rather lengthy period of change for some people — for some bodies, I should say. Truly, few will experience what we call the Keto Flu during the beginning of the diet, and it typically lasts about a week; so, don't be too concerned if you relate to these symptoms.

It occurs because the body is in a state similar to a shock from a drastic reduction to your regular carbohydrate intake. We have termed this kind of symptoms the Keto Flu because the symptoms are like standard influenza. For instance, some of the symptoms include nausea, headache, and weakness. If you feel any of these symptoms, you must be very careful to watch out for sugar cravings. This craving, on top of everything else, may make you feel miserable, and it could even possibly make you want to quit. However, there are ways to reduce these rather frustrating symptoms.

KETOSIS

Ketosis may seem like a scary word, but it is a completely natural metabolic state your body will enter when there is no longer glucose for your body to run off of. Instead, your body will begin to use fat as fuel! Exciting, right? Once your body has limited access to blood sugar or glucose, your body will enter a state of ketosis. You see, as you consume a low-carb diet, the levels of insulin hormones in your body will decrease, and the fatty acids in your body will be released from the fat stores.

From this point, the fatty acids that are being released in your body are then transferred to your liver. Once in place, the fatty acids are then oxidized and turned into ketone bodies which provide your body with energy. This process is important because the fatty acids cannot cross your blood-brain barrier, meaning they cannot provide energy to your brain (important). Once the process has occurred, ketones provide energy for your body and your brain without ever needing glucose.

Ketosis comes on anywhere from two days to one week after beginning the keto diet. This level is the goal of the keto diet to push your body into ketosis. Once you have reached a ketosis state, you will need to maintain the diet to remain in ketosis. Getting into ketosis is the worst side effect of the keto diet, but you will not regret your decision once you get past the initial stage. Ketosis is often referred to as keto flu because it feels much like you have viral flu. The symptoms of beginning ketosis are varied:

- Diarrhea

- Sleep disturbances

- Weakness during exercise and after

- Temporary loss of libido

- Exhaustion

- Cravings for sugary foods

- Headaches

- Bloating

- Irritability and moodiness

- Constipation

- Bad breath

The bad breath of ketosis is caused by waste products being eliminated from your body. These waste products are stored in fat cells and need to be eliminated as the fat cells are destroyed. Your body will eliminate waste through your breath, your sweat, or through defecation or urination.

You might naturally feel deprived of sugary treats when you begin the keto diet. We all love a good glazed doughnut or a massive bowl of cake and ice cream, and we miss these when they are gone. Just remember, they are not gone forever, and there is plenty of satisfying dessert options on the keto diet. You will crave carbs because they taste good, but you will be consuming enough foods not to need the carbs to make up for the caloric intake. And decreasing carb intake may lead to a decrease in your ability to sleep well at night. Consuming carbs causes the brain to release hormones melatonin and serotonin, which are the hormones that make you sleepy and happy, respectively. Eventually, the keto diet will teach your body to release hormones at the proper times, but in the meantime, try to keep a consistent sleep schedule even on your days off.

Some people will experience bloating, constipation, or diarrhea when beginning the keto diet. Food affects all people differently. Diarrhea comes from the increase in fats in your diet. The bloating is from the body releasing toxins from the stored fats that are being digested. Constipation may also go along with increased urination. Fat cells are the primary sources of water storage in your body. When you begin eliminating fat cells, the excess water leaves your body in the form of perspiration or urination, leaving very little for the bowels to use for defecation. And less water in your body may lead to feelings of fatigue or muscle weakness.

Moodiness and irritability come from the fact that you are now consuming fewer carbs than before. Carbs almost immediately turn into sugar when finished, whether the carb is a honey bun or a potato. The body does not care about the difference between healthy or unhealthy food; it just cares that food is coming in. Excess levels of sugar in the blood cause the body to release the hormones dopamine and serotonin, making you calm and happy. This hormone release is also why people often fall asleep after consuming a full of carbs. Removing these foods means that the brain will not signal the release of these hormones, and you might feel irritable or moody for a few days.

High-fat diets will increase the estrogen level in the woman's body because estrogen is stored in fat. Estrogen drives your desire for sex, and this is often lost during the first days of ketosis as all of those stored fat cells begin to disappear. When the body has eliminated enough stored fat and has already started functioning properly, the hormone levels will balance themselves . The estrogen production will return to normal, and your sex drive will reappear.

While these all might seem like good reasons to avoid the keto diet altogether, remember that these side effects are temporary. The beneficial effects of the keto diet are permanent. There are things that you can do to combat the symptoms of the keto flu and the beginning of ketosis to help you get through this period:

- Get a regularly scheduled seven to nine hours of sleep every night

- Engage in gentle exercises like walking, bicycling, or swimming

- Drink plenty of water to stay hydrated

- Add sea salt to your water to help ease muscle cramps. Lemon juice will help mask the saltiness

- Chew gum or suck sugar-free mints

Focusing on the positive benefits of the keto diet may also help you get through ketosis. The keto diet will naturally promote weight loss and assist you with managing your weight. The keto diet will easily incorporate into your everyday lifestyle. Fats and proteins will make you feel full for a more extended period, so you will eventually consume less food. Food cravings will disappear, and hunger will be eliminated. There is no need to count calories on the keto diet unless you are going for a specific weight loss goal. Keto will not slow down your metabolism, so you will continue to lose weight even after the first few weeks on a diet. You will feel more energetic and will be able to better focus on everyday tasks. Your muscles will become stronger and leaner.

Keto flu fades away, and you are left with the positive side effect of the keto diet which will last your entire lifetime. All bodies are different, and you may not see the same results that your neighbor might enjoy on the same diet plan. But follow the diet, eat the right foods, and you will be successful.

When you eat a low-carb, high-fat keto diet, your body will go into a state of ketosis, where it will switch from using carbohydrates and sugar as a source of energy to using ketones which act to burn the fat that you consume from the diet instead. To put your body into ketosis, you should ensure that you are eating fewer than 50 grams of carbohydrates each day.

The process of putting your body into a ketosis state does not happen immediately, and it can take a while before your body adapts to the changes. It can take two to seven days before your body goes into ketosis. The rate at which you go into ketosis depends on various factors including what your body type is, how many carbs you are eating each day, and how active you are.

You can decrease the time it takes for your body to go into ketosis by decreasing your carbohydrate intake to under 20 grams, supplementing certain nutrients in your diet, and doing intermittent fasting, where you only eat between certain times in the day.

So, how do I know if I am in ketosis, you ask? You will notice various indicators when your body has gone into ketosis, including weight loss, increased energy, reduced appetite, bad breath, improved focus and concentration, problems with your digestion like constipation and diarrhea, and not being able to sleep.

There are specialized ketone analyzer devices that you can buy that can help you monitor whether you are in ketosis or not. This is a great tool that you can use to give you accurate readings, although it can be quite pricey. You can use a blood ketone meter to measure the ketone levels in your blood; it is the most accurate form of testing you can perform. You can also use a ketone breath analyzer to measure the ketone levels in your breath. This method is not as accurate as testing your blood, but it is also still quite accurate.

Going into ketosis can have some adverse side effects, such as feeling tired, constipation, headache, bad breath, and increased levels of cholesterol, but these symptoms do not last throughout the entirety of the period that you are in ketosis, and these symptoms should go away after a while. After these initial symptoms, you will find that ketosis is relatively safe for your health and does not impact it negatively.

While staying in ketosis does not pose a problem to your health, you should come out of ketosis once you have reached your health and weight loss goals. It is recommended that you come out of ketosis every three months if you have not already come out of it sooner.

If your body goes out of ketosis before you have reached your health and weight loss goals, then you might not be following the keto diet in the right way, or you are including too many carbohydrates in your diet. When this happens, you can put your body back into ketosis by doing the same things you did the first time.

HOW TO MAINTAIN KETOSIS

This diet relies on you building a pattern that works for your body and your day-to-day activities. It will help a great deal if, when you do reach a ketogenic state, you can stay in it for a prolonged period. Fluctuating in and out of a ketogenic diet will exhaust you, and lead to you feeling that you cannot keep up. Therefore, you need to commit to maintaining ketosis. Ketosis should become a new normal for your body. Subsequently, you need to learn to identify when you are and are not in ketosis so that you can control the process.

First, you need to go into this diet aggressively. This is why it is important to be prepared, to make sure that you have all that you need to commit to the diet. Starting strong will cause a drastic change in the way your body functions. Therefore, you will be better able to notice the key signs of ketosis. If you were hoping to wean yourself slowly off of carbs, chuck this idea. Once you have started keto, you need to concern yourself with maintaining the momentum. Of course, this requires discipline. However, getting rid of the temptations in your pantry can help. Also, notice that the prescribed shopping lists contain a variety of delicious foods from which to choose: this should make your life better. The more variety, the less likely you are to get bored with the diet. So ensure that you create shopping lists with a lot of variety and buy products with many different flavors.

Testing your ketone level will also help you to maintain ketosis. It goes without saying that, when you know you are in it, you are more likely to maintain it. So, you might need to invest in ketone testing strips. Once you have used the strips long enough, you will be able to feel when you are or are not in ketosis; at this point, you can stop purchasing the strips.

Furthermore, tracking your macronutrient intake (as explained above) will ensure that you are in ketosis for longer periods. Obviously, if you are eating the correct ratio for your individual needs every day, you will be able to stay in ketosis longer. When you have a meal that is a little bit high on carbs, then you need to compensate by being active.

KETOSIS VS KETOACIDOSIS

When analyzing the difference between ketosis and ketoacidosis, it must be remembered that there are two completely different concepts. In fact, it is very easy and common to confuse these two terms, which are often misused as synonyms. This confusion may be caused by the fact that both are metabolic processes that involve the distribution of fat in the human body.

To clarify once and for all what must be distinguished between ketosis and ketoacidosis, the correct sequence must be followed. In the following, we first explain what they are and how they interfere with the body's metabolism. In addition, we will preview its relationship with nutrition and diabetes just to highlight their main characteristics.

WHAT IS KETOSIS?

As we saw in the previous topic, ketosis is a normal metabolic process caused by a high concentration of ketones in the blood (they are also called acetone). This phenomenon occurs when the body has used stored glycogen deposits and starts using and burning fat for energy. Lack of sugar due to minimal carbohydrate intake or fasting causes this immediate physiological reaction. The liver must produce more glucose, and hence the number of ketones entering the blood increases.

WHAT IS KETOACIDOSIS

Ketoacidosis commonly occurs in patients with type 1 diabetes, or those with type 2 in the final stage when their pancreas is no longer able to produce insulin. Diabetics should avoid and fasting carbohydrates in excessive quantities. Among the triggers of the development of ketoacidosis, the diseases whose symptoms present stages of high fever, vomiting, and diarrhea should be mentioned.

Other causes of ketoacidosis can be stress, physical or emotional trauma such as a heart attack. Alcohol and drug abuse can also trigger this disease. Some symptoms should make you aware of the risk of ketoacidosis: excessive thirst, frequent urination, abdominal pain, nausea and vomiting, shortness of breath, weakness or fatigue, mental confusion, and bad breath with a strong acetone odor.

DIFFERENCE BETWEEN KETOSIS AND KETOACIDOSIS

Under normal circumstances, ketones that enter the bloodstream are excreted through urine, sweat, and breath. The way the body carries out this process is the main difference between ketosis and ketoacidosis. In ketosis, the process of removing ketone bodies is natural and ongoing. This physiological process prevents the concentration of ketones in the blood.

In the case of ketoacidosis, ketone levels reach alarming levels and damage internal organs because the body can no longer metabolize ketones properly due to insufficient insulin production. If diabetes ketoacidosis is not treated on time, it can lead to further serious complications or even death. Diabetic ketoacidosis must be treated in a hospital by an experienced and competent team. If the reference structure does not contain a competent team, transferring to more suitable structures must be arranged.

In the case of ketoacidosis, a person with diabetes may have little appetite and little desire to eat. This can lead them to believe that it is better to reduce the dose of insulin. There is nothing left to prevent diabetic ketoacidosis, but it is important to strengthen blood sugar control and adjust the treatment regimen recommended by diabetes experts.

But how can the development of severe diabetic ketoacidosis be avoided? Diabetics need to measure their blood sugar levels regularly to stay in control. Your doctor (and family members) should also teach you how to recognize the symptoms of hyperglycemia beforehand so that you can respond quickly and go to the doctor immediately. A person with diabetes, who usually has a peak hyperglycemia, should be accustomed to regularly checking the body of ketones in the blood with the appropriate measuring tools.

THE RELATIONSHIP BETWEEN KETOSIS AND DIETS

The benefits you just saw make ketosis the basis of many diets. This diet plan reduces or completely eliminates carbohydrate consumption. Not surprisingly, most of these nutritional combinations are one of the main methods of weight loss. During ketosis, the body uses ketones instead of glucose to give cells what they need to produce energy. The immediate result is weight loss, but it has a side effect: the presence of different acetone in the blood. However, it must be remembered that the human body naturally has low levels of ketones in the blood; a limited amount that is not harmful to health.

Let's find out about ketoacidosis. Ketoacidosis is a pathological condition that occurs when blood sugar levels are high. The body cannot metabolize the amount of sugar properly due to a lack of insulin. With a sharp increase in ketones in the blood, severe abdominal pain and high levels of dehydration can occur. With such symptoms in mind, it is important to immediately go to the emergency room.

Unlike ketosis, ketoacidosis does not release ketones fast enough, and there is a risk that blood will radically increase its acidity. Changes to this sensitive condition can cause significant damage to the internal organs of the body. As you can see, this pathology is a serious condition that requires emergency treatment. In fact, if not treated properly, ketoacidosis can be fatal. An alarm signal is the smell of fruit or acetone which can be seen in a patient's breathing.

HOW TO IDENTIFY WHEN YOU ARE IN A STATE OF KETOSIS.

KETO BREATH

When you enter ketosis, your breath begins to smell noticeably. The breaking down of fats by your liver releases acetone. This acetone is responsible for the change in your breath. Keto breath smells fruity and/or metallic; many have likened it to the smell of overripe apples. You will find that you cannot get rid of the odor by brushing your teeth or using mouthwash. However, as the weeks progress, the smell will subside.

THIRST AND A DRY MOUTH

When your body is under ketosis, you will notice that you will become thirsty and experience a dry mouth. Under ketosis, your body has an increased need for water. You will also notice that you will urinate more and the urine will have a pungent smell.

APPETITE LOSS

The longer you adhere to the diet, the more opportunity you give your body to tap into your fat reserves for energy. Ultimately, this will result in decreased cravings for food. Your body will rely on your body's fat for sustenance, so you will not need to eat as much as you used to. This effect of the diet is quite helpful to the whole process because, if you are disciplined, your body will also come on board to help you succeed. You will also experience increased energy. Contrary to what you may be thinking, you will not feel starved and listless. You will realize that your mind functions better on this diet. You will have a clearer headspace, which will lead to a better mood.

BLOOD TESTS AND URINE TESTS

Blood and urine tests are the most accurate ways to detect whether you are in ketosis. The go-to test, however, is the urine test because it is inexpensive and you can do it at home. All you need to do is purchase the strips at a health store, dip a strip into a urine sample, and wait 15 seconds to get a color spectrum result. The spectrum will indicate how deep into ketosis you are. The darker the color, the deeper you are into ketosis.

CHAPTER 2
Benefits Ketogenic Diet

REDUCTION OF CRAVINGS AND APPETITE

Many people gain weight simply because they cannot control their cravings and appetite for caloric foods. The ketogenic diet helps eliminate these problems, but it does not mean that you will never be hungry or want to eat. You will feel hungry but only when you have to eat. Several studies have shown that the fewer carbohydrates you eat, the less you eat overall. Eating healthier foods that are high in fat helps reduce your appetite, as you lose more weight faster on a low-fat diet. The reason for this is that low carbohydrate diets help lower insulin levels as your body does not need too much insulin to convert glycogen to glucose while eliminating excess water in your body. This diet helps you reduce visceral fat. In this way, you will get a slimmer look and shape. It is the most difficult fat to lose, as it surrounds the organs as it increases. High doses can cause inflammation and insulin resistance. Coconut oil can produce an immediate source of energy as it increases ketone levels in your body.

REDUCTION OF RISK OF HEART DISEASE

Triglycerides, fat molecules in your body, have close links with heart disease. They are directly proportional as the more the number of triglycerides, the higher your chances of suffering from heart disease. You can reduce the number of free triglycerides in your body by reducing the number of carbohydrates, as is in the keto diets.

Over 647,000 people die from heart disease in America each year. Various factors can cause heart disease, such as inflammation in the arteries of the heart, diabetes, cholesterol, high blood pressure, heart defects, smoking, stress, obesity, and not following a well-structured diet.

By eating healthy fats and oils from the keto diet, such as olive oil, you can increase your high-density lipoprotein (HDL) cholesterol and lower your low-density lipoprotein (LDL). HDL is a type of cholesterol that is good for your body and helps to protect against LDL; the unhealthy type of cholesterol. When you eat fats and oils that are bad for you, LDL increases in your bloodstream and can build up in the walls of your arteries. When this happens, you can be at risk of heart disease. Healthy fats and oils help to reduce LDL and improve your heart health, lowering your risk of developing heart disease.

High blood pressure, otherwise known as hypertension, is one of the main causes of heart disease. When you have high blood pressure, your heart needs to work harder to pump the blood around your body, which can put a strain on your heart. Because of this, your heart can become damaged, and it can progress into heart disease. A low-carb diet can help you to normalize your blood pressure and lower your risk of heart damage and heart disease.

A low-carb, high-fat diet like keto can help you to lose excess weight, feel good about yourself, have lots of energy, and be able to make healthier decisions about your body and nutrition. Weight loss, an exercise routine, and a structured eating plan that caters to your needs as your body ages will help you to reduce your risk of heart disease and help to improve your symptoms if you have developed heart disease.

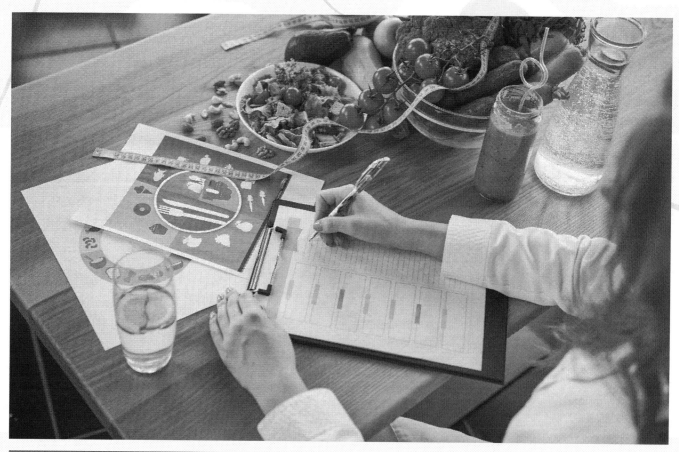

REDUCES CHANCES OF HAVING HIGH BLOOD PRESSURE

Weight loss and blood pressure have a close connection; thus, since you are losing weight while on the keto diet, it will affect your blood pressure.

FIGHTS TYPE 2 DIABETES

Type 2 diabetes develops as a result of insulin resistance. This is a result of having huge amounts of glucose in your system; with the keto diet, this is not a possibility due to the low carbohydrate intake.

Diabetes is a growing concern worldwide, with over 34 million people in the United States being diabetic. While a low-carb, high-fat diet like keto is not recommended for type 1 diabetics, it can be beneficial for those suffering from type 2 which helps to lower their blood glucose levels. The keto diet can be the healthiest lifestyle change that you can make to reduce your risk of developing type 2 diabetes and manage it effectively if you already suffer from it.

By reducing the number of calories that you consume each day in your diet, losing excess weight, and eating better food choices, you will be able to increase your body's sensitivity to insulin and reduce your blood sugar levels.

Many of the foods in the keto diet have a low glycemic load. This means that your blood sugar will not suddenly spike by eating these foods compared to if you ate foods that contain a high glycemic load. By eating foods with a low glycemic load, you can stabilize your blood sugar and reduce your body's need for insulin.

When you reduce your carbohydrates and increase your intake of fat, your body creates ketones to process these fats into a source of energy that your body can use throughout the day. The process that your body goes through to create these ketones helps to improve your response and resistance to insulin.

REDUCES RISK OF CANCER

The keto diet can help reduce your risk of developing cancer and is often used hand-in-hand with cancer treatment to help improve your symptoms if you are already suffering from cancer.

It has been found that some tumors grow larger and can spread in the presence of glucose sugar. By restricting carbohydrates and sugar in your diet, you can reduce the growth of these cancerous growths and stop them from spreading further.

If you are suffering from cancer, you should talk to your general practitioner or nutritionist before starting the keto diet so you can get their advice and they can potentially monitor your cancerous cell growth while you are on the keto diet.

IMPROVES BRAIN DISORDERS

The keto diet first came about as a diet to help treat children who were suffering from epilepsy and other brain disorders. Over the years, people have found that the keto diet can not only just work for children but also for people of all ages, including those in their 50s or older.

When carbohydrates and sugars are removed from a person's diet and their fat intake increases, their body is unable to use either as an energy source, and their body and brain uses ketones to burn the fat that they consume from their diet to give them energy throughout the day. When this happens, the person's brain receives energy from the ketones that are produced in their body and as a result, they experience fewer seizures.

The keto diet can also be beneficial to people who are suffering from Alzheimer's and Parkinson's disease. It has been shown that by eating a keto diet, you can decrease the symptoms associated with Alzheimer's disease and stop it from getting worse. Symptoms of Parkinson's disease can also be improved with the keto diet.

IMPROVES SYMPTOMS OF PCOS

Polycystic ovary syndrome (PCOS) is a health condition whereby a woman's body produces more male hormones than it normally should. When this happens, you might experience irregular or skipped periods, and you will have problems with getting pregnant. If you have PCOS, you have a higher risk of heart disease and developing type 2 diabetes.

When you eat foods that contain carbohydrates and sugar, your insulin levels increase. When your insulin levels are high and you suffer from PCOS, your ovaries produce male hormones like testosterone, which in turn can cause your periods to become more irregular and cause you to grow more body hair.

By following a low-carb, high-fat keto diet, your insulin levels will remain steady and, as a result, your ovaries will not produce more male hormones in your body than it needs. This allows your period to become more regular and helps to improve other symptoms related to PCOS that you might be experiencing.

IMPROVES SYMPTOMS OF METABOLIC SYNDROME

When you are at risk of developing type 2 diabetes and heart disease, you will experience symptoms called metabolic syndrome, which include gaining weight around your stomach area, your levels of "good" HDL cholesterol have decreased and your "bad" LDL cholesterol has increased, high blood pressure, high blood sugar levels, and an increased amount of triglycerides in your blood.

By following a low-carb, high-fat keto diet, you will be able to treat and even reverse these symptoms and improve your quality of life by decreasing your risk of developing type 2 diabetes and heart disease. The keto diet can help you to lose stomach weight, improve your levels of "good" HDL cholesterol, stabilize your blood pressure and blood sugar levels, and decrease triglycerides in your blood.

INCREASES THE PRODUCTION OF HDL

High-density lipoprotein is referred to as good cholesterol. It is responsible for caring calories to your liver, thus can be reused. High fat and low carbohydrate diets increase the production of HDL in your body, which also reduces your chances of getting heart disease. Low-density lipoprotein is referred to as bad cholesterol.

SUPPRESSES YOUR APPETITE

It is a strange but true effect of the keto diet. It was thought that this was a result of the production of ketones, but this was proven wrong as a study taken between people on a regular balanced diet and some on the keto diet and their appetites were generally the same. It, however, helps to suppress appetite as it has a higher fat content than many other diets. Food stays in the stomach for longer as fat and is digested slowly, thus provides a sense of fullness. On top of that, proteins promote the secretion of cholecystokinin, which is a hormone that aids in regulating appetite. It is also believed that the ketogenic diet helps to suppress your appetite by continuous blunting of appetite. There is increased appetite in the initial stages of the diet, which decreases over time.

CHANGES IN CHOLESTEROL LEVELS

This is kind of on the fence between good and bad. This is because the ketogenic diet involves a high fat intake, which makes people wonder about the effect on blood lipids and its potential to increase the chances of heart disease and strokes, among others. Several major components play a lead role in determining this, which are: LDL, HDL, and blood triglyceride levels. Heart disease correlates with high levels of LDL and cholesterol. On the other hand, high levels of HDL are seen as protection from diseases caused by cholesterol levels. The impacts of the diet on cholesterol are not properly known. Some research has shown that there is no change in cholesterol levels while others have said that there is change. If you stay in deep ketosis for a very long time, your blood lipids will increase, but you will have to go through some negative effects of the ketogenic diet which will be corrected when the diet is over. If a person does not remain following the diet strictly for like ten years, he/she will not experience any cholesterol problems. It is difficult to differentiate the difference between diet and weight loss in general. The effect of the ketogenic diet on cholesterol has been boiled down to if you lose fat on the ketogenic diet, then your cholesterol levels will go down, and if you don't lose fat, then your cholesterol levels will go up. Strangely, women have a larger cholesterol level addition than men while both are on a diet. As there is no absolute conclusion on the effect of the ketogenic diet on cholesterol, you are advised to have your blood lipid levels constantly checked for any bad effects. Blood lipid levels should be checked before starting the diet and about eight weeks after starting. If repeated results show a worsening of lipid levels, then you should abandon the diet or substitute saturated fats with unsaturated fats.

BALANCE HORMONES AND BOOST ENERGY

If you have been experiencing difficulty with balancing your hormones, especially if you are going through menopause, you know how cumbersome these side effects can be. From hot flashes to mood swings, you have likely experienced it all in a very short time. This can become very discouraging because it can often feel that nothing helps the symptoms. Many women who are presently going through this have started to try Keto as a desperate attempt to make a difference, and they are finding that it does, indeed, help level things out. Even if your symptoms are very bad, Keto has been shown to lessen them and make your life feel easier again.

It works so well because of the increase in fat consumption. While you have likely never been encouraged to consume more fat in any previous diet plan you've been on, Keto allows you to do this because it is literally changing the way that your body stores and breaks down this fat. When your body has more of these good fats inside, it will be prompted to create more estrogen and progesterone. This shows that, when you start a diet that slashes your fat consumption, you might actually be causing this hormonal imbalance to become more severe without even realizing it.

For those still dealing with periods, Keto helps by detoxifying the body. PMS symptoms are lessened when the body reaches this point of detoxification. PMS can become very hard to deal with because it produces an excess of estrogen. When you have too much estrogen in your system, this is when you will begin to feel cramping, bloating, and mood swings that you have been dealing with for years. This estrogen dominance can occur more severely in certain cases when your diet consists of too many sugary foods. What you need is additional progesterone to balance you out. Because the Keto diet detoxifies you, it will be getting rid of the excess hormones that you don't need and begin to replace them with the ones that you are lacking.

LOW ENERGY LEVELS

When available, the body prefers to use carbohydrates for fuel as they burn more effectively than fats. General drop-in energy level is a concern raised by many dieters due to the lack of carbohydrates. Studies have shown that it causes orthostatic hypotension which causes lightheadedness. It has come to be known that these effects can be avoided by providing enough supplemental nutrients like sodium. Many of the symptoms can be prevented by providing 5 grams of sodium per day. Most times, fatigue disappears after a few weeks or even days, if fatigue doesn't disappear, then you should add a small number of carbohydrates to the diet as long as ketosis is maintained. The diet is not recommended when caring out high-intensity workouts, weight training, or high-intensity aerobic exercise as carbohydrates are an absolute requirement, but it is okay for low-intensity exercise.

EFFECTS ON THE BRAIN

It causes increased use of ketones by the brain. The increased use of ketones, among other reasons, result in the treating of childhood epilepsy. As a result of the changes that occur, the concern over the side effects, including permanent brain damage and short-term memory loss, has been raised. The origin of these concerns is difficult to understand. The brain is powered by ketones in the absence of glucose. Ketones are normal energy sources and not toxic as the brain creates enzymes, during fetal growth, that help us use them. Epileptic children, though not the perfect examples, show some insight into the effects of the diet on the brain in the long term. There is no negative effect in terms of cognitive function. There is no assurance that the diet cannot have long-term dietary effects, but no information proves that there are any negative effects. Some people feel they can concentrate more when on the ketogenic diet, while others feel nothing but fatigue. This is as a result of differences in individual physiology. There are very few studies that vaguely address the point on short-term memory loss. This wore off with the continuation of the study.

CONSTIPATION

A common side effect of the diet is reduced bowel movements and constipation. This arises from two different causes: lack of fiber and gastrointestinal absorption of foods. First, the lack of carbs in the diet means that, unless supplements are taken, fiber intake is low. Fiber is very important to our systems. High fiber intake can prevent some health conditions, including heart disease and some forms of cancer. Use some type of sugar-free fiber supplement to prevent any health problems and help you maintain regular bowel movements. The diet also reduces the volume of stool due to enhanced absorption and digestion of food; thus, fewer waste products are generated.

FAT REGAIN

Dieting, in general, has very low long-term success rates. There are some effects of getting out of a ketogenic diet like the regain of fat lost through calorific restriction alone. This is true for any diet based on calorific restrictions. It is expected for weight to be regained after carb reintroduction. For people who use the weighing scale to measure their success, they may completely shun carbs as they think it is the main reason for the weight regain. You should understand that most of the initial weight gain is water and glycogen.

IMMUNE SYSTEM

There is a large variety in the immunity system response to ketogenic diets on different people. There has been some repost on reduction on some ailments, such allergies and increased minor sickness susceptibility.

OPTIC NEUROPATHY

This is optic nerve dysfunction. It has appeared in a few cases, but it is still existence. It was linked to the people not getting adequate amounts of calcium or vitamin supplements for about a year. All the cases were corrected by supplementation of adequate vitamin B, especially thiamine.

THE TRANSITION IS HARD

All the benefits we listed above start happening once you're in ketosis, but while you're getting there, it can be a really difficult transition. A lot of people experience the "keto flu," which is essentially withdrawal from carbs. The more carbs you're used to, the worse the withdrawal is. Symptoms include nausea, headaches, and irritability. It can be hard to predict how bad you'll feel or how long the transition will take. Many people don't want to put themselves through such an unpleasant experience. One solution is to transition slowly by gradually cutting out carbs. You'll just have to wait longer to enter ketosis and start seeing benefits.

IT'S TOO RESTRICTIVE TO BE PRACTICAL FOR THE LONG-TERM

There are a lot of foods you can't eat on the ketogenic diet, and it can be difficult to avoid those ingredients. A lot of people follow the diet for a short time as a way to "reset" their health, but in the long-term, going keto can be really hard. An eating lifestyle that's so restrictive can be emotionally taxing and lead to cheating, which can throw you out of ketosis. What's the point if that happens? It can be tempting to go back to unhealthy eating habits because the keto diet is so demanding.

TOO MANY KETONES HAVE NEGATIVE CONSEQUENCES

You can have too much of a good thing on the ketogenic diet. A high number of ketones actually makes your blood more acidic, which causes a condition known as ketoacidosis. For diabetics, this can be fatal if untreated. Symptoms include stomach pains, nausea, vomiting, and dehydration. Acidic blood damages your kidneys and liver if you don't do anything about it. That's why that range of 1.5 - 3 mmol/L (and just 1.5 mmol/L for diabetics) is important to maintain.

IT ELIMINATES TOO MANY NUTRIENTS

Nutritionists aren't very fond of the keto diet because of the foods it eliminates. There are lots of important vitamins and minerals you don't get from their best sources, and it can lead to what's known as micronutrient deficiency. If you aren't careful to fill in those gaps with other foods or supplements, you can miss out on sodium, magnesium, and potassium. Not getting enough of these nutrients will result in dehydration, headaches, nausea, low energy, weak bones, and so on.

YOUR BODY WILL HAVE A CHANGED PERIOD

It depends from person to person on the number of days that will be, but when you start any new diet or exercise routine, your body has to adjust to the new normal. With the keto diet, you are drastically cutting your carbohydrate intake, so the body has to adjust to that. You may feel slow, weak, fatigued, and like you are not thinking as quickly or fast as you used to. It just means your body is adjusting to keto and once this change period is done, you will see the weight loss results you expected.

IF YOU ARE AN ATHLETE, YOU MAY NEED MORE CARBOHYDRATES

If you still want to try keto as an athlete, it's important you talk to your nutritionist or trainer to see how the diet can be tweaked for you. Most athletes require a greater intake of carbs than the keto diet requires, which means they may have to up their intake to assure they have the energy for their training sessions. High endurance sports (like rugby or soccer) and heavy weightlifting require a greater intake of carbohydrates. If you're an athlete wanting to follow keto and gain the health benefits, it's important you first talk to your trainer before changing your diet.

YOU HAVE TO CAREFULLY COUNT YOUR DAILY MACROS

For beginners, this can be tough, and even people already on keto can become lazy about this. People are often used to eating what they want without worrying about just how many grams of protein or carbs it contains. With keto, be meticulous about counting your intake to ensure you are maintaining the keto breakdown (75% fat, 20% protein, ~5% carbs). The closer you stick to this, the better results you will see regarding weight loss and other health benefits. If your weight loss has stalled or you're not feeling as energetic as you hoped, it could be because your macros are off. Find a free calorie counting app and be sure you look at the ingredients of everything you're eating and cooking.

CHAPTER 3
Getting Started on Keto After 50

When you are over 50, you will need to look at different changes that occur in the body. These changes will determine the quality of life that you will live in. Making dietary changes is an essential aspect that can go a long way in boosting your youthfulness. You will lose unwanted weight without the need to step into a gym. The keto diet has proven to be effective for people with a background of health issues such as obesity, blood sugar issues, and those who are suffering from emotional eating. Before we go into more details about the keto diet, we should get some background information about it.

You have already done much of the work to change over to a healthy lifestyle now that you know how Keto works. Of course, to make the most of the knowledge, you still have a lot to learn.

While the previous chapter gave you the theoretical side of Keto, this one tells you how to take action on the information you have. You'll also learn some of the common mistakes new Keto followers make and how to avoid them.

You'll learn how to be proactive in your approach by keeping a log of your daily eating habits. Your Keto journal will make sure you are making real progress.

Before we cover the common mistakes women make with Keto, first, we need to look a little deeper into Ketosis itself. As you know, practitioners of this diet are doing it as a way to trigger Ketosis.

Ketosis is the biological process in which your liver produces Ketones that cause your body to burn fat for energy. You get this to happen by depriving your body of its usual source of energy: carbs.

But it is actually a little more complicated than that, despite what other Keto books might have you believe. This is a way of explaining Ketosis that understandably simplifies it, but by doing so, it ignores some of the important components of Ketosis.

First of all, it isn't quite true that your body burns carbs for energy. Instead, your body uses those carbs to burn something else for energy: glucose. Glucose is the sugar that comes from the food that you eat.

It is different from the sugar you have in your pantry. Your digestive system breaks down everything you eat into its most basic parts so it can use the food for energy. Glucose is what comes out of this process of digestion. You could say it is the basic source of energy for your body.

When you put your body through Ketosis, this is a way of getting your system to use ketones for the job that carbs would normally do. Meanwhile, the ketones themselves get your body to burn more fat.

What makes Keto attractive to many women is the fact that it uses biological mechanisms already present in your body to burn fat. You aren't taking a pill to lose weight that won't actually work. Your body can already go through ketosis without any medication; all you have to do is follow the Keto diet.

It isn't exactly true when people say you put your body through ketosis to get these ketones to burn fat. The job of ketones is not to burn fat, but to aid in the process of burning through glucose.

When you don't eat a lot of carbs, carbs don't do the job of burning your glucose anymore. Instead, your liver produces ketones that burn fat.

There is a lot of misinformation that spreads because people learn about Keto from word-of-mouth or other unreliable sources instead of learning about it directly from a book.

Many people get the false impression that the only thing we do in Keto is lower our carb intake. They do not think there is any more to it than that. Of course, it is a major part of Keto. But if it is the only part of the Keto diet you are following, you are not going about it healthily.

That's because the other vitally important aspect of the Ketogenic diet is eating healthy fats. Make sure you get that into your mind because it is extremely important.

If you aren't getting a lot of healthy fats into your diet, and you aren't eating many carbs, you are not doing Keto. This is simply bad for your body. When you eat few carbs, you are already depriving your body of something it normally has, putting your cells in a state of stress that will trigger autophagy while simultaneously — and most importantly — triggering Ketosis.

Ketosis will indeed cause an influx of ketones that burn through your fat. However, if you don't have healthy fats to burn for energy, you will end up hurting yourself.

Everyone needs energy to live. Someone who deprives themselves of carbs and fats will only end up hurting themselves. When you dramatically decrease your carb intake in Keto, make sure you replace those calories with healthy, nutrient-rich foods like vegetables and sources of healthy fats.

By this point, you will experience the subjective changes that come with changing to a Keto lifestyle. You will feel a surge of energy, notice significant weight loss, and even feel cleansed through the natural process of autophagy. You will notice all of these things as long as you closely follow the directions provided here.

However, you may be looking for a more tangible way of seeing your progress in Keto. There is a way you can figure out how strong your Ketosis is, and all it requires is a blood sugar tester.

This may not be for everyone. For some people, the subjective difference they feel in their energy and the weight loss itself will be enough for them to know they are in Ketosis. They might not like the idea of having to draw blood to test their Ketosis with the blood sugar tester. Maybe the price of the blood sugar tester isn't worth it; it isn't exactly expensive, but it isn't exactly cheap, either. This is completely fine; if you feel like you are getting what you need from Keto, that should be enough for you.

Others want to know for a fact that Ketosis is the reason for their weight loss. They want to be certain that their other lifestyle changes are not the reason for their weight loss.

There is a method for you to be more certain if you are going through significant Ketosis. You just need a blood sugar tester to calculate your glucose-ketone index.

The Ketone-glucose index will tell you whether you are going through significant Ketosis. It will also indicate whether you are going through advanced autophagy.

First, purchase the blood sugar tester. After that, you want to wait until you have been following Keto for a long enough time. I recommend waiting until you have been on Keto for two weeks. If you have only been doing Keto for a week, this test will not be accurate.

In fact, you will want to be sure you have been consistently doing Keto for two weeks — without cheating the requirements — before taking this blood sugar test. Only then should you take the results seriously.

After you are on Keto for two weeks, you will plug the numbers from the test into a specific formula. This formula will give you your glucose-ketone index. The meter will give you a numeral for glucose and another for ketone.

For blood sugar meters that use mmol/L, as most do, you will have to divide the glucose numeral by 18. You will not have to divide by 18 if the blood sugar test uses mg/dL because this part of the equation is only to get us to use the correct units.

Once the conversion is done, the next thing you do is divide your glucose value by the ketone value. You can remember which is which from the name of the index: glucose-ketone. Start with your glucose and divide it by your ketone. After that, you will have your glucose-ketone index. It is as simple as that. From there, it is only a matter of interpreting this number and knowing what it means.

As a general rule, you would like a glucose-ketone index from 6 to 9. This indicates that your body is going through significant Ketosis. Now let's talk about where you definitely don't want to fall on the glucose-ketone index. If your index is lower than 3, this is where you may be going through some stage of cancer and may even experience seizures.

Of course, you won't be in this range of the index unless you already know you have cancer or some other serious condition, so this isn't something you need to think much about.

On the less extreme end of things, if your glucose-ketone index goes from 3 to 6, that is an indicator that you suffer from obesity. It is unlikely that you will have an index in this range if you are only overweight, especially on the lower end.

If you are overweight and not obese, and you find yourself on the lower end of this 3 to 6 range, you may be in danger of slipping from the overweight territory into obesity, so keep that in mind.

This is certainly not where you want to land when you put yourself through Ketosis, but that doesn't mean you aren't going through Ketosis in this range. The glucose-ketone index may be the most objective metric we have, but there are a lot of different factors that can come into play.

If you are already overweight and follow the Keto diet consistently and correctly for two weeks, you may still be somewhere in the 3 to 6 range. You may just have to wait until you lose some more weight before you see your index increase and go above 6.

An index above 9 is not desirable; it simply means you are not going through significant Ketosis. You will have to stick with it longer to see this number drop.

Ultimately, you want your index to fall somewhere between 6 and 9. For a woman seeking to trigger Ketosis, this is the ideal index to have. Since this index tells you that you are going through significant Ketosis, it comes with a lot of good news. When you fall within this range, you will find it relatively easy to maintain the weight you have or lose weight if you aren't content with where you are.

As I said, you need to look at this index with some skepticism. Just because it is the most tangible way to look at the progression of your Ketosis, that doesn't make it perfect. Even if your index is between 6 and 9, that doesn't mean you should blindly accept that to mean you are going through Ketosis. Unfortunately, it just isn't that easy.

You should look for subjective signs as well as your index to determine if your Ketosis is significant.

These signs include the health of your skin, whether you are losing weight, and how much energy you feel you have every day.

In the same way, an index outside of 6 and 9 doesn't mean you definitely are not going through Ketosis. With the many factors that go into it, it could just be the last thing you ate.

The reason for the variability is because blood sugar fluctuates a lot. Your blood sugar level at one moment won't be the same as the blood sugar level you have at the next.

When you use the index, use it together with some plain common sense. Ask yourself if you feel better, whether your skin looks better, and look at the number on the scale. These will all be as useful as the index.

Don't look at the glucose-ketone index as the only way of measuring how healthy you are. You could fall between 6 and 9 and not be healthy. If you fall outside 6 and 9 from time to time, you might still be healthy, too. You should take all of these things into consideration.

Finally, I suggest you keep a journal with all of this information in it. Mark down the days you go to the gym, what exercises you do, and how much time you spend there. Mark down what Keto-friendly foods you are eating, and write down their carb, fat, protein, and calorie content.

Chapter six goes through 100 + recipes you can follow, so you have a month's worth of foods that all fit into the Keto diet. I am positive you will love eating these delicious meals.

WHY KETO FOR 50+?

For instance, indigestion becomes common as you age. This happens because the body is not able to break down certain foods as well as it used to. With all of the additives and fillers, we all become used to putting our bodies through discomfort in an attempt to digest regular meals. You are probably not even aware that you are doing this to your body; but upon trying a Keto diet, you will realize how your digestion will begin to change. You will no longer feel bloated or uncomfortable after you eat. If you notice this as a common feeling, you are likely not eating food that is nutritious enough to satisfy your needs and is only resulting in excess calories.

Keto fills you up in all of the ways that you need, allowing your body to truly digest and metabolize all of the nutrients. When you eat your meals, you should not feel the need to overeat to overcompensate for not having enough nutrients. Anything that takes stress off of any system in your body is going to become a form of anti-aging. You will quickly find this benefit once you start your Keto journey as it is one of the first-reported changes that most participants notice. In addition to a healthier digestive system, you will also experience more regular bathroom usage, with little to none of the problems often associated with age.

While weight loss is one of the more common desires for most 50+ women who start a diet plan, the way that the weight is lost matters. If you have ever shed a lot of weight before, you have probably experienced the adverse effects of sagging or drooping skin that you were left to deal with. Keto actually rejuvenates the elasticity in your skin. This means that you will be able to lose weight and your skin will be able to catch up. Instead of having to do copious amounts of exercise to firm up your skin, it should already be becoming firmer each day that you are on the Keto diet. This is something that a lot of participants are pleasantly surprised to find out.

Women also commonly report a natural reduction in wrinkles, and healthier skin and hair growth, in general. Many women who start the diet report that they actually notice reverse effects in their aging process. While the skin becomes healthier and more supple, it also becomes firmer. Even if you aren't presently losing weight, you will still be able to appreciate the effects that Keto brings to your skin and face. Because your internal systems are becoming healthier by the day, this tends to show on the outside in a short amount of time. You will also begin to feel healthier. While it is possible to read about the experiences of others, there is nothing like feeling this for yourself when you begin Keto.

Everyone, especially women over 50, has day-to-day tasks that are draining and require certain amounts of energy to complete. Aging can, unfortunately, take away from your energy reserve, even if you get enough sleep at night. It limits the way that you have to live your life, and this can become a very frustrating realization. Most diet plans bring about a sluggish feeling that you are simply supposed to get used to, for example. But Keto does the exact opposite. When you change your eating habits to fit the Keto guidelines, you are going to be hit with a boost of energy. Since your body is truly getting everything that it needs nutritionally, it will repay you with a sustained energy supply.

Another common complaint about women over 50 is that seemingly overnight, your blood sugar levels are going to be more sensitive than usual. While it is important that everyone keeps an eye on these levels, it is especially important for those who are in their 50s and beyond. High blood sugar can be an indication that diabetes is on the way, but Keto can become a preventative measure that we've already talked about. Additionally, naturally regulating elevated blood sugar levels also reduces systemic inflammation, which is also common for women over 50. By balancing the immune system, of which inflammation is part, common aches and pains are reduced. If, for example, you've noticed that you have been feeling stiff lately, even despite your efforts to exercise and stretching, this is likely due to a normal case of inflamed joints. Inflammation can also affect vital organs and is a precursor to cancer. Keto will support your path to an anti-inflammatory lifestyle.

Sugar is never great for us, but it turns out that sugar can become especially dangerous as we age. What is known as a "sugar sag" can occur when you get older because the excess sugar molecules will attach themselves to the skin and protein in your body. This doesn't even necessarily happen because you are eating too much sugar. Average levels of sugar intake can also lead to this sagging as the sugar weakens the strength of your proteins that are supposed to hold you together. With sagging comes even more wrinkles and arterial stiffening.

If you have any anti-aging concerns, the Keto diet will likely be able to address your worries. It is a diet that works extremely hard while allowing you a fairly simple and direct guideline to follow in return. While your motivation is necessary to form a successful relationship with Keto, you won't need to worry about doing anything "wrong," or accidentally breaking from your diet. As long as you know how to give up your sugary foods and drinks while making sure that you are consuming the correct amount of carbs, you will be able to find your own success while on the diet.

TIPS FOR KETO DIET FOR WOMEN OVER 50

Keto Tip number one that is so important is DRINK WATER! This is absolutely vital for any diet that you are on, and you need it if not on one as well. However, this vital tip is crucial on a keto diet because when you are eating fewer carbs, you are storing less water, meaning that you are going to get dehydrated very easily. You should aim for more than the daily amount of water; however, remember that drinking too much water can be fatal as your kidneys can only handle so much at once. While this has mostly happened to soldiers in the military, it does happen to dieters as well, so it is something to be aware of.

Along with that same tip is to keep your electrolytes. You have three major electrolytes in your body. When you are on a keto diet, your body is reducing the amount of water that you store. It can be flushing out the electrolytes that your body needs as well, and this can make you sick. Some of the ways that you can fight this are by either salting your food or drinking bone broth. You can also eat pickled vegetables.

Eat when your hungry instead of snacking or eating constantly. This is also going to help, and when you focus on natural foods and healthy foods, this will help you even more. Eating processed foods is the worst thing you can do for fighting cravings, so you should really get into the routine of trying to eat whole foods instead.

Another routine that you can get into is setting a note somewhere that you can see it that will remind you of why you're doing this in the first place and why it's important to you. Dieting is hard, and you will have moments of weakness where you're wondering why you are doing this. Having a reminder will help you feel better, and it can really help with your perspective.

Tracking progress is something that straddles the fence. A lot of people say that this helps a lot and you can celebrate your wins; however, as everyone is different and they have different goals, progress can be slower in some than others. This can cause others to be frustrated and sad, as well as wanting to give up. One of the most important things to remember is that while progress takes time, you shouldn't get discouraged if you don't see results right away. With most diets, it takes at least a month to see any results. So, don't get discouraged and keep trying if your body is saying that you can. If you can't, then you will need to talk to your doctor and see if something else is for you.

You should make it a daily routine to try and lower your stress. Stress will not allow you to get into ketosis, which is the state that keto wants to put you in. The reason for this being that stress increases the hormone known as cortisol in your blood, and it will prevent your body from being able to burn fats for energy. This is because your body has too much sugar in your blood. If you're going through a really high period of stress right now in your life, then this diet is not a great idea. Some great ideas for this would be getting into the habit or routine of taking the time to do something relaxing, such as walking and making sure that you're getting enough sleep, which leads to the next routine that you need to do.

You need to get enough sleep. This is so important not just for your diet, but also for your mind and body as well. Poor sleep also raises those stress hormones that can cause issues for you, so you need to get into the routine of getting seven hours of sleep at night on the minimum, and nine hours if you can. If you're getting less than this, you need to change the routine you have in place right now and make sure that you establish a new routine where you are getting more sleep. As a result, your health and diet will be better.

Another routine that you need to get into is to give up diet soda and sugar substitutes. This is going to help you with your diet as well because diet soda can actually increase your sugar levels to a bad amount, and most diet sodas contain aspartame. This can be a carcinogen, so it's actually quite dangerous. Another downside is that using these sugar substitutes just makes you want more sugar later. Instead, you need to get into the habit of drinking water or sparkling water if you like carbonation.

Staying consistent is another routine that you need to get yourself into. No matter what you are choosing to do, make sure it's something that you can actually do. Try a routine for a couple of weeks and make serious notes of mental and physical problems that you're going through, as well as any emotional issues that come your way. Make changes as necessary until you find something that works well for you and that you can stick to. Remember that you need to give yourself time to get used to this and time to get used to changes before you give up on them.

Be honest with yourself as well. This is another big tip for this diet. If you're not honest with yourself, this isn't going to work. Another reason that you need to be honest with yourself is if something isn't working, you need to be able to understand that and change it. Are you giving yourself enough time to make changes? Are you pushing too hard? If so, you need to understand what is going on with yourself and how you need to deal with the changes that you're going through. Remember not to get upset or frustrated. This diet takes time, and you need to be able to be a little more patient to make this work effectively.

Getting into the routine of cooking for yourself is also going to help you so much on this diet. Eating out is fun, but honestly, on this diet, it can be hard to eat out. It is possible to do so with a little bit of special ordering and creativity, but you can avoid all the trouble by simply cooking for yourself. It saves time, and it saves a lot of cash.

Getting into the routine of having snacks on hand is a good idea as well. This keeps you from giving in to temptation while your out, and you can avoid reaching for that junk food. You can make sure that they are healthy, and you will be sticking to your high-intensity diet, which is what you want. There are many different keto snacks that you can use for yourself to eat.

A good tip would be to use keto sticks or a glucose meter. This will give you feedback on whether your users do this diet right. The best option here is a glucose meter. It's expensive, but it's the most accurate. Be aware that if you use ketostix; they are cheaper, but the downside is that they are not accurate enough to help you. A perfect example is that they have a habit of telling people their ketone count is low when they are actually the opposite.

Try not to overeat as this will throw you out of where you need to be. Get into the routine of paying attention to what your eating and how much. If this is something that you're struggling with, try investing in a food scale. You will be able to see exactly what it is your eating and make sure that you are understanding your portions and making sure you stay in ketosis.

Another tip is to make sure that you're improving your gut health. This is so important. Your gut is pretty much linked to every other system in your body, so make sure that this something that you want to take seriously. When you have healthy gut flora, your body's hormones, along with your insulin sensitivity and metabolic flexibility will all be more efficient. When your flexibility is functioning at an optimal level, your body can adapt to your diet easier. If it's not, then it will convert the fat your trying to use for energy into body fat.

Batch cooking or meal prepping is another routine that is a good thing to get into. This is an especially good routine for on-the-go women. When you cook in batches, you can -make sure that you have meals that are ready to go, and you don't have to cook every single day, in that way, you can save a lot of time as well. You will also be making your environment better for your diet because you're supporting your goals instead of working against them.

The last tip is to mention exercise again. Getting into the routine of exercising can boost your ketone levels, and it can help you with your issues transitioning to keto. Exercises also use different types of energy for your fuel that you need. When your body gets rid of the glycogen storages, it needs other forms of energy, and it will turn into that energy that you need. Just remember to avoid exercises that are going to hurt you. Stay with the smaller exercises and lower intensity.

Following these tips and getting into these routines is going to help you stay on track and make sure that your diet will go as smoothly as it possibly can.

ADDITIONAL TIPS

EAT A LOT OF HIGH FIBER VEGETABLES

Fresh vegetables contain innumerable substances that the body needs for its vital functions. Vegetables include fiber, vitamins, minerals, and a range of phytonutrients that regulate the metabolism. According to some studies conducted by the University of Minnesota in 2012, phytonutrients "work as antioxidants, phytoestrogens and anti-inflammatory agents." Make sure to eat vegetables of different colors with each meal.

CHOOSE CLEAN FATS AND SUPPORT THE INTESTINES

In addition to minimizing carbohydrates, increasing the consumption of good healthy fats is really the basis of any ketogenic diet plan. Organic linseed oil, evening primrose oil, avocado oil, and coconut oil are all excellent options. Also, you can consume foods such as wild salmon, raw walnuts, seeds, and avocados. Of course, the extra virgin olive oil is also perfect. Healthy fats that contain Omega 3, such as those just described, can reduce inflammation in the intestine, and promote the growth of good intestinal bacteria. If you were a big carbohydrate consumer before you started, your gut will probably be a little tried. You must then help it with prebiotic or probiotic foods.

By following the keto diet, hormones are rebalanced; those specific hormones that are specifically designed to regulate the sense of hunger. If you are used to eating too much or, conversely, not eating enough, try eating by noticing when you feel completely satisfied and full. If you are not sure, slow down while you eat and wait a few minutes between mouthfuls.

INCLUDE INTERMITTENT FASTING

Intermittent fasting is often an integral part of any ketogenic diet plan. Typically, a person is required to refrain from eating solid food for 14-18 hours, and this sets in motion a whole host of powerful healing mechanisms. One of these processes is cellular autophagy or the fact that old cells die and are replaced by new ones. However, if you feel dizzy or nauseated, you should stop fasting and eat something immediately.

AVOID INFLAMMATORY FOODS

By eliminating sugar and gluten in high-carbohydrate foods, you can reduce your own level of inflammation. However, there may be other foods that cause inflammation, like milk and milk products.

STAY WELL HYDRATED

Our body consists mainly of water. Fluid is responsible for several important functions in the body, including digestion and circulation. Drink enough water to maintain muscle mass, intestinal health, and increase detoxification. Several studies have shown that a 1% decrease in hydration is enough to negatively affect mood, attention, motor skills, and even memory.

Move

Long sitting or lying down hurts long-term health. On the other hand, many studies have shown a link between moderate but constant exercise and reduced inflammation, and better immune function.

KEEP AN EYE ON STRESS

The Ketogenic diet works well as long as you keep stress at bay. Chronic stress actually produces excessive hormones, including cortisol, which keeps the body awake and in a condition of inflammation. What can you do every day to reduce stress? Meditation, breathing exercises, natural walks, or several minutes of stretching.

TAKE CARE OF YOUR BODY

Each individual is his own world and must be taken into account. Every day you have to ask yourself the following questions: How do I feel today? Am I feeling mentally stable? Am I focused? It should also be remembered that each body reacts differently, especially in the first phase of the keto diet. To take care of your body, all you have to do is "adjust" how you feel at a particular moment and what your body needs at that moment. As you might have noticed, eliminating totally carbohydrates is not enough to get good results even if you don't go on the ketogenic diet. Finally, I advise you, as always, to rely on an experienced nutritionist to adjust your diet and find out if it is appropriate to follow the ketogenic option.

Learn to minimize your consumption of carbohydrates; to achieve ketosis, the most important is doing away with high-carb diets. When you minimize your intake of carbohydrates, your body is forced to burn its fats as a way of replacing the glucose that would normally be used to energize your body. This way, your body is bound to achieve ketosis.

Learn to increase your fats intake healthily; by now, you already know that consuming an increased level of healthy fats could improve the ketone levels in your body, as well as help your body reach ketosis. You could also opt to choose from a variety of animal and plant fats to improve your ketone levels in the body.

Learn to fast; by fasting, you significantly improve your body's chances of reaching ketosis. You could decide to go for hours without eating. Fasting has been proven to quickly get your body into ketosis.

Learn to test your ketone levels and make the right adjustments; this is important because it will give you a chance to know if the diet is working effectively or if adjustments are needed. It is important to test your ketone levels to determine how your body is fairing.

Learn to regulate your protein consumption; for your body to reach ketosis, you have to ensure that your consumption of proteins is regulated, not excessively consumed, but adequately consumed.

Learn to put your body in an active state; you could decide to engage your body in physical activities such as jogging, swimming, hiking, playing basketball or football, or going to the gym. This is important because your body's ketone levels improve when your body is in an active state. You could speed up this process by fasting and working out at the same time.

KEEPING YOURSELF INSPIRED

It is important to seek out inspiration with everything that you do in life. Having a source of inspiration will provide you with even more motivation to reach your goals. In a way, this guide can serve as your first source of inspiration as you begin your Keto journey. By reading about the facts and benefits of the lifestyle, you should feel excited and ready to begin. Once you get the hang of Keto, you will start to become your own inspiration. You can do so by being persistent with your routine.

Everyone has routines that they follow throughout the day, whether they change frequently or remain the same. Having routines means that you have a sense of stability, which is great! Your routine should be regular enough to keep you on track, yet flexible enough to never become boring or stale. A great routine has room for mistakes and plenty of room for changes, if necessary.

Each morning recite some positive affirmations to yourself as you begin your day. These affirmations can be as simple as "I can do this," or as complex as you want them to be. No matter what is going on in your life, if you start the day with positivity, you are likely going to be able to return to this positivity later on. Use your breakfast time as a chance for you to enjoy the fact that you are nourishing your body. No matter what you are eating, any Keto breakfast is going to prepare you for the day ahead. If you are bringing lunch with you to work, make sure that it is packed and ready to go with you. Without having to struggle to decide what you'd like to eat for lunch that day, you are taking away one stressor. The more stressors that you can eliminate, the better your day will go.

Remember to savor your lunch once you get the chance to eat it. Sit down and enjoy your food. Let the quality and healing properties of the food inspire you. Your lunch break should be used for eating and nothing else. If you are multitasking during this time, your body isn't going to reach a state of relaxation. All of the tension and stress that you have been holding onto throughout the morning is going to follow you as you eat your lunch. This can cause your digestive system to act up, potentially even causing you indigestion or an upset stomach. Stress tends to build up in your stomach which can definitely influence your appetite. Know that, no matter what is going on around you, you'll be able to return to it after you enjoy your lunch. It's amazing what a few moments of relaxation can do to break up all of the different elements that you have been experiencing throughout your day.

If you do find an opportunity to eat out with your friends, take this as a personal challenge of your knowledge about the Keto diet. Think about any substitution that can be made to classic restaurant food. Know that you shouldn't be ashamed that you are focused on your health. Being on a diet isn't the end of your fun and happiness. It is meant to become a regular part of your lifestyle. Your friends and loved ones should also be understanding and supportive of your cause. If you show them that the Keto diet is making you feel great, then there is no reason why the ones who care about you the most would make you feel guilty for being on the diet. Your support system is very important during this time, so make sure that you are aware of the company that you are keeping. A good support system should be an inspirational, encouraging, and supportive voice while you are on your journey. You might even find that they will become interested in trying out the diet for themselves.

As you have been learning about the Keto diet for yourself, you have likely been able to see past many of the stigmas that people talk about. This happens with nearly any diet plan because dieting has been a controversial topic in society for the last several decades. By spreading accurate information about the Keto diet and being a living example of someone who is on it, you are doing your best to educate those around you. When you can show people that you aren't actually "starving" and that you are receiving benefits such as weight loss and energy boosts, this can truly change minds about how the Keto diet really works. People are going to be naturally skeptical, but as long as you stay true to what you know, you will be able to continue seeing the successful results that you desire.

Let dinner time be your chance to explore new options. Whether you are eating in with the family or going out to a new restaurant, try to have something new for dinner each night to keep you intrigued with the diet. There are so many options for what you can make given the ingredients that Keto boosts. You will always have a protein-packed entree that is full of flavor. Because you can cook with butter and oil, all of your favorite dishes can be replicated without having to skip over them. People truly enjoy how many of their favorite savory meals are included in the guidelines of the Keto diet. Some people say that it almost feels too good to be true that they are still able to eat these things! Eating healthy, healing foods is definitely a source of inspiration.

When you take the time to make sure that your body feels great by exercising, know that this is a reason to be inspired by yourself and your choices. It can be difficult to get up and moving, especially while on a new diet. Commend yourself for the effort that you put into your workout routines and know that, paired with the Keto diet, you are going to be seeing results very soon. When you get into these habits, you will be more likely to return to them again in the future on your own. They become less like tasks to complete and more like normal parts of your day that you can expect. When you get into the full swing of Keto, it should feel natural and effortless.

MOST COMMON MISTAKES AND HOW TO FIX THEM

Do you feel like you are giving your all to the keto diet, but you still aren't seeing the results you want? You are measuring ketones, working out, and counting your macros, but you still aren't losing the weight you want. Here are the most common mistakes that most people make when beginning the keto diet.

TOO MANY SNACKS

There are many snacks you can enjoy while following the keto diet, like nuts, avocado, seeds, and cheese. But snacking can be an easy way to get too many calories into the diet while giving your body an easy fuel source besides stored fat. Snacks need to be only used if you frequently hunger between meals. If you aren't extremely hungry, let your body turn to your stored fat for its fuel between meals instead of dietary fat.

NOT CONSUMING ENOUGH FAT

The ketogenic diet isn't all about low carbs. It's also about high fats. You need to be getting about 75 percent of your calories from healthy fats, 5 percent from carbs, and 20 percent from protein. Fat makes you feel fuller longer, so if you eat the correct amount, you will minimize your carb cravings, and this will help you stay in ketosis. This will help your body burn fat faster.

CONSUMING EXCESSIVE CALORIES

You may hear people say you can eat what you want on the keto diet as long as it is high in fat. Even though we want that to be true, it is very misleading. Healthy fats need to make up the biggest part of your diet. If you eat more calories than what you are burning, you will gain weight, no matter what you eat because these excess calories get stored as fat. An average adult only needs about 2,000 calories each day, but this will vary based on many factors like activity level, height, and gender.

CONSUMING A LOT OF DAIRIES

For many people, dairy can cause inflammation and keeps them from losing weight. Dairy is a combo food, meaning it has carbs, protein, and fats. If you eat a lot of cheese as a snack for the fat content, you are also getting a dose of carbs and protein with that fat. Many people can tolerate dairy, but moderation is the key. Stick with no more than one to two ounces of cheese or cream at each meal. Remember to factor in the protein content.

CONSUMING A LOT OF PROTEIN

The biggest mistake that most people make when just beginning the keto diet is consuming too much protein. Excess protein gets converted into glucose in the body called gluconeogenesis. This is a natural process where the body converts the energy from fats and proteins into glucose when glucose isn't available. When following a ketogenic diet, gluconeogenesis happens at different rates to keep body function. Our bodies don't need a lot of carbs, but we do need glucose. You can eat absolute zero carbs, and through gluconeogenesis, your body will convert other substances into glucose to be used as fuel. This is why carbs only make up five percent of your macros. Some parts of our bodies need carbs to survive, like kidneys, medulla, and red blood cells. With gluconeogenesis, our bodies make and stores extra glucose as glycogen just in case supplies become too low.

In a normal diet, when carbs are always available, gluconeogenesis happens slowly because the need for glucose is extremely low. Our body runs on glucose and will store excess protein and carbs as fat.

It does take time for our bodies to switch from using glucose to burning fats. Once you are in ketosis, your body will use fat as the main fuel source and will start to store excess protein as glycogen.

NOT GETTING ENOUGH WATER

Water is crucial for your body. Water is needed for all your body does, and this includes burning fat. If you don't drink enough water, it can cause your metabolism to slow down, and this can halt your weight loss. Drinking 64 ounces or one-half gallon every day will help your body burn fat, flush out toxins, and circulate nutrients. When you are just beginning the keto diet, you might need to drink more water since your body will begin to get rid of body fat by flushing it out through urine.

CONSUMING TOO MANY SWEETS

Some people might indulge in keto brownies and keto cookies that are full of sugar substitutes just because their net carb content is low, but you have to remember that you are still eating calories. Eating sweets might increase your carb cravings. Keto sweets are great on occasion; they don't need to be a staple in the diet.

NOT GETTING ENOUGH SLEEP

Getting plenty of sleep is needed to lose weight effectively. Without the right amount of sleep, your body will feel stressed, and this could result in your metabolism slowing down. It might cause it to store fat instead of burning fat. When you feel tired, you are more tempted to drink more lattes for energy, eat a snack to give you an extra boost, or order takeout rather than cooking a healthy meal. Try to get between seven and nine hours of sleep each night. Understand that your body uses that time to burn fat without you even lifting a finger.

LOW ON ELECTROLYTES

Most people will experience the keto flu when they begin this diet. This happens for two reasons. When your body changes from burning carbs to burning fat, your brain might not have enough energy, and this, in turn, can cause grogginess, headaches, and nausea. You could be dehydrated, and your electrolytes might be low since the keto diet causes you to urinate often.

Getting the keto flu is a great sign that you are heading in the right direction. You can lessen these symptoms by drinking more water or taking supplements that will balance your electrolytes.

CONSUMING HIDDEN CARBS

Many foods look like they are low carb, but they aren't. You can find carbs in salad dressings, sauces, and condiments. Be sure to check nutrition labels before you try new foods to make sure it doesn't have any hidden sugar or carbs. It just takes a few seconds to skim the label, and it might be the difference between whether or not you'll lose weight.

If you have successfully ruled out all of the above, but you still aren't losing weight, you might need to talk with your doctor to make sure you don't have any health problems that could be preventing your weight loss. This can be frustrating but stick with it. Stay positive and stay in the game. When the keto diet is done correctly, it is one of the best ways to lose weight.

Getting energy from fat, not sugar, is a very good approach and, as we have seen, can bring various health benefits. However, if you keep on the ketogenic diet every day, you can make some mistakes. If you know them, you can avoid them and realize their full potential.

GIVE UP BEFORE YOU STOP KETOSIS

Food ketosis is a mandatory step and has more or less obvious and more or less long-term effects. They vary depending on how much carbohydrate has been abused before and how much our hearts are overloaded. When the body switches from burning sugar to burning fat, we feel like poisoned and weighed. They are poisons that rise and start blooming again after one or two weeks. Other symptoms associated with persistent ketosis include:

- Halitosis

- A little nauseous

- Early hunger for sugar

- Fatigue

- Nervousness

- A little sadness

These last symptoms are related to the effects of sugar and carbohydrate excretion on our mind, which makes us happy and satisfied by stimulating the same opiate receptors.

Conversely, if you stop them now and lose the allure, you might feel a little sad and nervous.

Many are afraid of these symptoms and are not well informed. They believe that the ketogenic diet is not for them, that they are worse off at the start and give up everything before they switch to ketosis.

LACK OF SALT AND MINERALS

The desire for sugar, which was originally accused, can be exacerbated by the possibility of mineral deficiencies. Therefore, they need to be integrated with the right dose of potassium, magnesium, and sodium. Using Himalayan salt, eating salty snacks, using magnesium in the evening, could be just as many ways to remedy this mistake.

CONSUME BAD QUALITY FOOD

It is another of the most common mistakes. We focus on weight loss, but continue to consume frozen, canned, highly processed, and, as mentioned, proteins that are practical and quick to eat, but of poor quality.

DO NOT INTRODUCE THE RIGHT AMOUNT OF FIBER

Vegetables should always be fresh and consumed in twice the amount of protein and always cooked intelligently; that is, never subjected to overcooking or too high temperatures. In everyday life, if present, however, we often resort to ready-made, frozen, or packaged vegetables. Also concerning fruit, we often resort to the very sugary one, we forget that there are many berries with a low glycemic index: berries, mulberries, goji berries, Inca berries, maqui.

CONSUME THE HIGHEST PROTEIN LOAD AT DINNER

This is a mistake that involuntarily we all commit. The work, the thousand commitments, lead us to stay out all day, to eat a frugal meal for lunch, or even not to consume it at all. Here, the dinner turns into the only moment of the day in which we find our family members, we have more time, we are more relaxed, and we finally allow ourselves a real meal complete with vegetables, proteins, sometimes even carbohydrates and then fruit or dessert to finish. It escapes us that even the healthiest protein, the freshest or most organic food, weighs down the liver. During the night, this being busy helping digestion, it cannot perform the other precious task: to purify the blood, prepare hormones, energy for the next day.

CHAPTER 4
Foods to Eat & Avoid in Keto Diet

FOODS TO AVOID

For us women over 50 who want to get into the Keto diet, it is good to know the foods that we should avoid, like grains, fruits with high sugar content, starchy vegetables, fruit juice and carrot juice, sugar (including honey and syrup), chips, crackers, and baked goods. These items are high in sugar and carbohydrates and will not be useful in a low-carbohydrate Keto diet.

FRUITS AND STARCHY VEGETABLES

Juice, fruit, and sugar are definite no-no's on the keto diet. The excess sugars will not only spike your carbohydrates, but they will also cause insulin to be released in response to the spike in blood sugar. It is all the opposite of the goal of ketosis. There will be too many carbohydrates available for the body to convert to energy. It will make it impossible for the body to be starved of carbs and glucose, and the body will not switch to using fat as energy. Starchy vegetables like corn and beets have high sugar content. Bananas, apples, raisins, and mangoes are too high in sugar content to include on the keto diet. Fruit and sugar will have to be avoided to reach ketosis.

GRAINS, BREAD, AND PASTA

Grains are high in carbohydrates. Don't try to substitute grains with gluten-free bread and pasta. Even gluten-free items tend to replace the grains with other foods that are also high in carbohydrates like chickpea flour.

To replace pasta, try the zucchini spirals or shirataki noodles. These noodles are very low in carbohydrates and may be an alternative to high-carb grain pasta that meets your needs. Butternut squash spirals are also readily available, but winter squash is high in carbohydrates. Quinoa is a protein-rich grain; there are too many carbohydrates for this grain to be included in the keto food list. Rice and potatoes, brown rice, and sweet potatoes have too many carbs for even the healthy alternatives to be included in your food plan.

LEGUMES

Avoid beans and legumes like lentils, pinto, black beans, and chickpeas. Though they happen to be high in fiber, they unfortunately also are high in carbohydrates. That makes beans a poor addition to the ketogenic diet. They can be used sparingly when added in small amounts to recipes like soups and stews. They are nutritious, but like starchy vegetables, they do not fit well in the keto lifestyle.

COATED MEAT

Meats with added sugar such as flavored maple sausage and bacon should be avoided. Also, breaded chicken and fish are not allowed on the keto diet. These foods have carbohydrates and are not options on the diet. It is better to eat less processed food, and if there are any added flavorings, you should add them yourself to maintain control of the additions.

LOW FAT

Foods labeled as low fat often contain sugar or unapproved sugar substitutes which act like sugar and trick your body into a spike in blood sugar and short-term satisfaction. It is right for items you may not associate with sweet flavors like salad dressing and mayonnaise. In these instances, full-fat options are included on the keto diet, so it's okay to eat real food and avoid processed imitation.

VEGETABLE OILS

The nutritional value of vegetables, canola, and corn oils is not ideal for the keto diet since they are high in polyunsaturated fatty acids (PUFA). These PUFAs are bad for your heart as they release plaque into arteries. They also cause inflammation in the liver and may promote liver disease. Vegetable oils may be a cause of obesity. Vegetable oils are unhealthy.

Of course, most foods are technically allowed on the ketogenic diet. To include some of these forbidden foods in your diet and remain in ketosis, measure your foods and flavorings and know what you are consuming when it comes to carbohydrates and overall calories. Because carbohydrates' consumption spikes blood sugar levels, when blood sugar drops, there will be a feeling of malaise and hunger when the carbohydrates wear off. It is better to eat more calories from foods that will sustain a constant blood sugar level and foods to help keep your stomach feeling full.

FOODS ALLOWED IN KETO DIET

To make the most of your diet, there are prohibited foods and others that are allowed but in limited quantities. Here are the foods allowed in the ketogenic diet:

LEAN OR FATTY MEATS

No matter which meat you choose, it contains no carbohydrates, so you can have fun! Pay attention to the quality of your meat, and the amount of fat. Alternate between fatty meats and lean meats!

Here are some examples of lean meats:

- Beef: sirloin steak, roast beef, 5% minced steak, roast, flank steak, tenderloin, grisons meat, tripe, kidneys

- Horse: roti, steak

- Veal: cutlet, shank, tenderloin, sweetbread, liver

- Chicken and turkey: cutlet, skinless thigh, ham

- Rabbit

Here are some examples of fatty meats:

- Lamb: leg, ribs, brain

- Beef: minced steak 10, 15, 20%, ribs, rib steak, tongue, marrow

- Pork: ribs, brain, dry ham, black pudding, white pudding, bacon, terrine, rillettes, salami, sausage, sausages, and merguez

- Veal: roast, paupiette, marrow, brain, tongue, dumplings

- Chicken and turkey: thigh with skin

- Guinea fowl

- Capon

- Turkey

- Goose: foie gras

LEAN OR FATTY FISH

The fish does not contain carbohydrates so you can consume unlimited! As with meat, there are lean fish and fatty fish, pay attention to the amount of fat you eat and remember to vary your intake of fish. Oily fish have the advantage of containing a lot of good cholesterol, so it is beneficial for protection against cardiovascular disease! It will be advisable to consume fatty fish more than lean fish to be able to manage your protein intake: if you consume lean fish, you will have a significant protein intake and little lipids, whereas, with fatty fish, you will have a balanced protein and fat intake!

Here are some examples of lean fish:

- Cod
- Colin
- Sea bream
- Whiting
- Sole
- Turbot
- Limor career
- Location
- Pike
- Ray

Here are some examples of oily fish:

- Swordfish
- Salmon
- Tuna
- Trout
- Monkfish
- Herring
- Mackerel
- Sardine

EGGS

Eggs contain no carbohydrates, so you can consume as much as you want. It is often said that eggs are full of cholesterol and that you have to limit their intake, but the more cholesterol you eat, the less your body will produce by itself! In addition, it's not just poor-quality cholesterol, so you can consume 6 per week without risk! And if you want to eat more but you are afraid of your cholesterol and I have not convinced you, remove the yellow!

Egg yolks are rich in healthy cholesterol, which could be essential in reducing your chances of contracting heart diseases. Eggs are also rich in other nutrients, which could be important in ensuring your eyes are well maintained.

VEGETABLES AND RAW VEGETABLES

Yes, you can eat vegetables. But you have to be careful which ones: you can eat leafy vegetables (salad, spinach, kale, red cabbage, Chinese cabbage...) and flower vegetables (cauliflower, broccoli, Romanesco cabbage...), as well as avocado, cucumbers, zucchini or leeks, which do not contain many carbohydrates.

FRESH CHEESES AND PLAIN YOGURTS

Consume with moderation because they contain carbohydrates.

NUTS AND OILSEEDS

They have low levels of carbohydrates but are rich in saturated fatty acids, that's why they should moderate their consumption. Choose almonds, hazelnuts, Brazil nuts, or pecans.

COCONUT (IN OIL, CREAM, OR MILK)

It contains saturated fatty acids, that's why we limit its consumption. Cream and coconut oil contain a lot of medium-chain triglycerides (MCTs), which increase the level of ketones, essential to stay in ketosis.

BERRIES AND RED FRUITS

They contain carbohydrates in reasonable quantities, but you should not abuse them to avoid ketosis (blueberries, blackberries, raspberries...).

KETOGENIC BEVERAGES

Foods high in carbs are not recommended for the Ketogenic Diet. This also applies to drinks and beverages. Drinks that have high levels of carbs should be avoided. Soda, coffee drinks, or iced tea are some of the drinks that you should abstain from. In simpler terms, all drinks that you intend to ingest must be in line with the requirements of the Ketogenic diet. Furthermore, avoid all sugar-sweetened drinks, fruit juice included because they have sugar, which constitutes the consumption of carbs. Traces of carbs are also found in dairy milk omitting milk as Keto-friendly.

In the meantime, water, green tea (unsweetened), sparkling water (a good replacement for soda once you consider ditching soda a challenge), unsweetened coffee, bone broth, and nut milk are Keto-friendly drinks you could opt to use.

HEALTHY KETOGENIC SNACKS

Almost all the snacks that first come to mind are high in carbs and thus are not Keto-friendly. This could be very frustrating if you have just started on the diet and you find yourself hungry in between meals, and the need to replenish yourself is overwhelming. Worry not! This book will certainly cater to that need. These are some of the snacks that you could consume to replenish your body in the case that you get hungry between meals for several reasons and you would need to feed again. The following snacks are all Keto-friendly;

- Fatty meat and fish (meatball slides)

- Strawberries and cream

- Guacamole with vegetable sticks

- Low carbohydrates milkshake with almond milk, nutritional berries, and cocoa which is the powder form

- Cheese

- Cheese with olives

- Boiled eggs

- Small portions of leftover meals

- Dark chocolate (90%)

- Ketogenic smoothies

- Fermented vegetables, including fermented cabbage, cauliflower, green beans, beets, carrots, or cucumbers.

- Buffalo cauliflower bites served with blue cheese and carrot sticks.

- Coconut yogurt is an alternative to regular or traditional yogurt.

- Ground flax seeds accompanied by cheese.

- Mix nuts including almonds, pecans, Brazil nuts, cashew, walnuts, and pistachios.

- Avocado usage in the place of mayonnaise while consuming the egg salad.

- Sushi rolls that support the Ketogenic diet.

- Mix mayonnaise with cooked salmon and have a salad that is Keto friendly

EATING OUT ON A KETOGENIC DIET

You could find yourself working late in the office or stuck in traffic for long periods, and you could start to wonder if you would have the time to prepare yourself a Ketogenic meal. You may not have the time to prepare yourself that meal and end up being forced to dine in a restaurant. Worry not! These tips will guide you on what to eat in diners or restaurants and still maintain your Ketogenic diet meal plan.

It is actually very easy to make most of the meals served in restaurants Keto-friendly when you are dining out. You could combine a few foods and end up eating a Keto-friendly meal.

You could eat egg-based meals in the restaurant, such as omelet or bacon, which support the Ketogenic Diet and still maintain your body on ketosis perfectly well.

Replacing the high-carb foods with lots of vegetables is another good option, or you could decide to order the bun-less burger and replace the fries with green vegetables to go with cheese and avocado.

As for dessert, you could opt to order berries with cream or order for a mixed cheese board.

It is recommended that while dining out, you should serve a meal with either meat, fish, or any egg-based dish, as well as ingest vegetables instead of high-carb foods and having cheese for dessert. It takes time before you can fully master how to dine out and still be on your Keto meal plan. This means you should be easy on yourself and learn as time goes by.

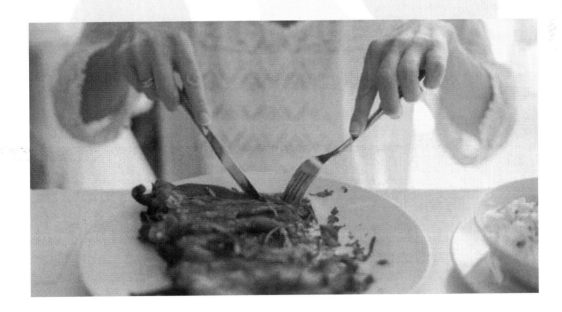

CHAPTER 5
Keto Diet 28-days meal plan

WEEK 1

MONDAY

Breakfast: Detox Tea

Lunch: Ham and Cheese Keto Stromboli

Dinner: Easy Chicken Cordon Bleu Casserole

Snack: Oven-baked Bacon Chips

TUESDAY

Breakfast: Egg White Spinach Omelet

Lunch: Prosciutto, Caramelized Onion, & Parmesan Braid

Dinner: Low-Carb Keto Indian Butter Chicken

Snack: Grain-Free Amaretto Cookies

WEDNESDAY

Breakfast: Bacon Frittata

Lunch: Spaghetti Squash with Meatballs

Dinner: Cheese Fathead Pizza Crust

Snack: Keto Guacamole

THURSDAY

Breakfast: Cheese & Onion Quiche

Lunch: Easy Shrimp Avocado Salad with Tomatoes

Dinner: Beef Chili Recipe (Beanless Chili)

Snack: Keto Fudge Brownies

FRIDAY

Breakfast: Cheese & Onion Quiche

Lunch: Baked Grill Chicken with Feta and Dill

Dinner: Easy Keto Bacon Cheeseburger Skillet.

Snack: Grain-Free Amaretto Cookies

SATURDAY

Breakfast: Keto French Toast

Lunch: Air Fryer Turkey Meatballs

Snack: Eggs of any style and coffee with heavy cream without any carb sweetener.

Dinner: Keto chocolate Greek yogurt cookies and Keto beef and sausage balls

SUNDAY

Breakfast: Keto cauliflower and eggs with keto coffee

Lunch: Keto burger and Keto creamy granola

Dinner: Tomato Chili Chicken Tender with Fresh Basils

Snacks: Keto pizza and Tangerine avocado smoothie

SHOPPING LIST

- Cheese
- Meat
- Turkey
- Eggs
- Chicken
- Pork
- Chocolate
- Amarettos
- Coffee

- Avocado
- Shrimp
- Tomatoes
- Spinach
- Parsley
- Garlic
- Bacon
- Onions
- Cheese, butter,

- cream, and milk
- Butter
- Cheddar cheese
- Almond milk
- Heavy cream
- Greek yogurt

MONDAY

Breakfast: Homemade Sage Sausage Patties

Lunch: Cheddar Broccoli Soup

Dinner: Keto Bacon Cheeseburger Casserole

Snack: Keto Low Carb Lemon Blueberry Bread

TUESDAY

Breakfast: Cinnamon Roll Cereal

Lunch: Avocado Tuna Melt Bites

Dinner: Italian Cheese Stuffed Meatloaf

Snack: Healthy Avocado Chocolate Cookies

WEDNESDAY

Breakfast: Eggs Florentine Casserole

Lunch: Homemade Keto Caesar Salad

Dinner: Keto Jalapeno Popper Stuffed Chicken

Snack: Keto Fermented Dill Pickles

THURSDAY

Breakfast: Keto Breakfast Grits

Lunch: Grilled Tuna Salad with Garlic Dressing

Dinner: Keto Chicken Parmesan

Snack: Buffalo Cauliflower Bites

FRIDAY

Breakfast: Keto Mushroom Omelet

Lunch: Keto Cloud Bread

Dinner: Keto Ham and Cheese Crustless Quiche

Snack: Keto Crackers

SATURDAY

Breakfast: Keto Lemon Chia Pudding

Lunch: Ketofied Chick-Fil-A Chicken

Dinner: Keto Garlic Dusted Dinner Rolls

Snack: Garlic Bacon Dip

SUNDAY

Breakfast: Keto Crepes

Lunch: Keto Roasted Pumpkin & Halloumi Salad

Dinner: Keto One Skillet Chicken in Lemon Cream Sauce

Snack: Chicken Skin Crisps with Spicy Avocado Cream (Fat Bombs)

SHOPPING LIST

- Cauliflower
- Avocado
- Pumpkin
- Mushroom
- Ham
- Lemon
- Chia
- Chicken
- Bacon
- Sausage

- Broccoli
- Eggs
- Chicken
- Beef
- Tuna
- Garlic
- Tomatoes
- Garlic
- Onions
- Cauliflower

- Avocado
- Oregano
- Jalapeños
- Cheese, butter, cream, and milk
- Butter
- Cheddar cheese
- Almond milk
- Yogurt
- Chocolate

WEEK 3

MONDAY

Breakfast: Keto Eggs Benedict

Lunch: Keto Meaty Mediterranean Lunch Bowls

Dinner: Keto Mexican Zucchini and Beef

Snack: Cheesy Meatballs

TUESDAY

Breakfast: Keto Granola Cereal

Lunch: Keto Crispy Ginger Mackerel Lunch Bowl

Dinner: Hamburger Sausage and Broccoli Alfredo

Snack: Mediterranean Roll-Ups (Fat Bombs)

WEDNESDAY

Breakfast: Keto Meal Replacement Shake

Lunch: Keto Bacon Cheeseburger Kebabs

Dinner: Keto Cauliflower Pizza Crust

Snack: Buffalo Chicken Fingers

THURSDAY

Breakfast: Huevos Rancheros

Lunch: Keto Tuna Cheese Melt

Dinner: Bacon Cheeseburger Soup

Snack: Chorizo-Stuffed Jalapenos

FRIDAY

Breakfast: Keto Breakfast Enchiladas

Lunch: Keto Thai Fish Curry

Dinner: Lasagna Stuffed Portobellos

Snack: Onion Rings

SATURDAY

Breakfast: Keto Chicken and Waffle Sandwiches

Lunch: Creamy Keto Fish Casserole

Dinner: Pesto Spinach Artichoke Chicken Bake

Snack: Peanut Butter Power Granola

SUNDAY

Breakfast: Keto Pepperoni Pizza Quiche

Lunch: Keto Meat Pie

Dinner: Bacon Ranch Chicken Crust Pizza

Snack: Keto Brownie Bark

SHOPPING LIST

- Eggs
- Chicken
- Spinach
- Granola
- Turkey breast
- Beef
- Peanut Butter
- Deli ham

- Pork
- Anchovy fillets
- Fruits and vegetables:
- Tomatoes
- Spinach
- Parsley
- Garlic
- Onions

- Broccoli
- Red cabbage
- Cheese, butter, cream, and milk
- Butter
- Cheddar cheese
- Almond milk
- Muenster cheese
- Heavy cream

MONDAY
Breakfast: Gooey Keto Cinnamon Rolls
Lunch: Keto Lasagna
Dinner: Moroccan Meatballs
Snack: Coconut Chocolate Chip Cookies — Low Carb and Gluten-Free

TUESDAY
Breakfast: Keto Lemon Sugar Poppy Seed Scones
Lunch: Keto Asian Cabbage Stir-Fry
Dinner: Keto Tacos
Snack: Classic Blueberry Scones

WEDNESDAY
Breakfast: Bacon Kale and Tomato Frittata
Lunch: Italian Keto Meatballs with Mozzarella Cheese
Dinner: Low Carb Big Mac Bites
Snack: Classic Chocolate Cake Donuts

THURSDAY
Breakfast: Vegan Keto Scramble
Lunch: Easy Low-Carb Cauliflower Mac 'n Cheese
Dinner: Keto Fried Chicken in the Air Fryer
Snack: Homemade Caramel Frappuccino

FRIDAY
Breakfast: Keto Sausage Gravy and Biscuit Bake
Lunch: Cobb Salad
Dinner: Keto Easy Herb-Roasted Turkey
Snack: Homemade Graham Crackers

SATURDAY
Breakfast: No-tatoes Bubble and Squeak
Lunch: Keto Instant Pot Soup (Low Carb)
Dinner: Pork Fried Rice
Snack: Keto Cinnamon Roll Biscotti

SUNDAY
Breakfast: Lemon Raspberry Sweet Rolls
Lunch: Easy Keto Beef Tacos

Dinner: Roast Pork Belly

Snack: Raspberry Lemonade Smoothies

SHOPPING LIST

- Chocolate
- Rice
- Meat
- Eggs
- Raspberry
- Chicken
- Biscotti
- Beef
- Fruits and vegetables:
- Tomatoes

- Kales
- Cauliflower
- Avocado
- Sausages
- Cheese, butter, cream, and milk
- Parmesan cheese
- Mozzarella cheese
- Butter
- Cheddar cheese
- Muenster cheese

- Heavy cream
- Grass-fed butter

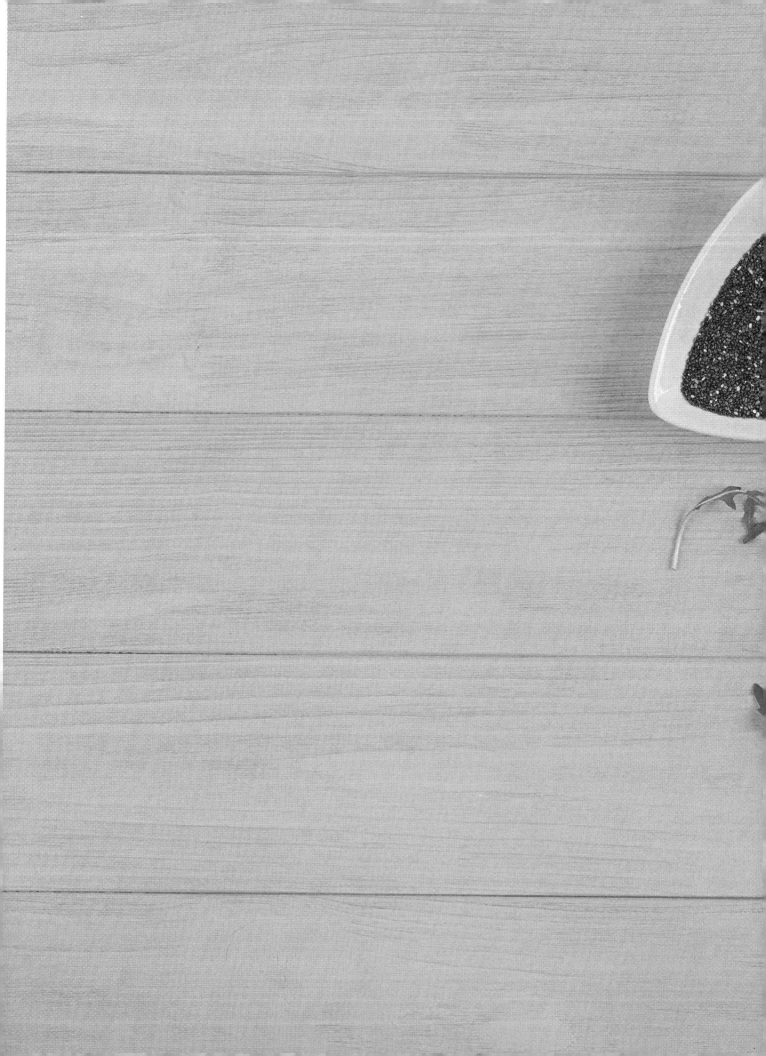

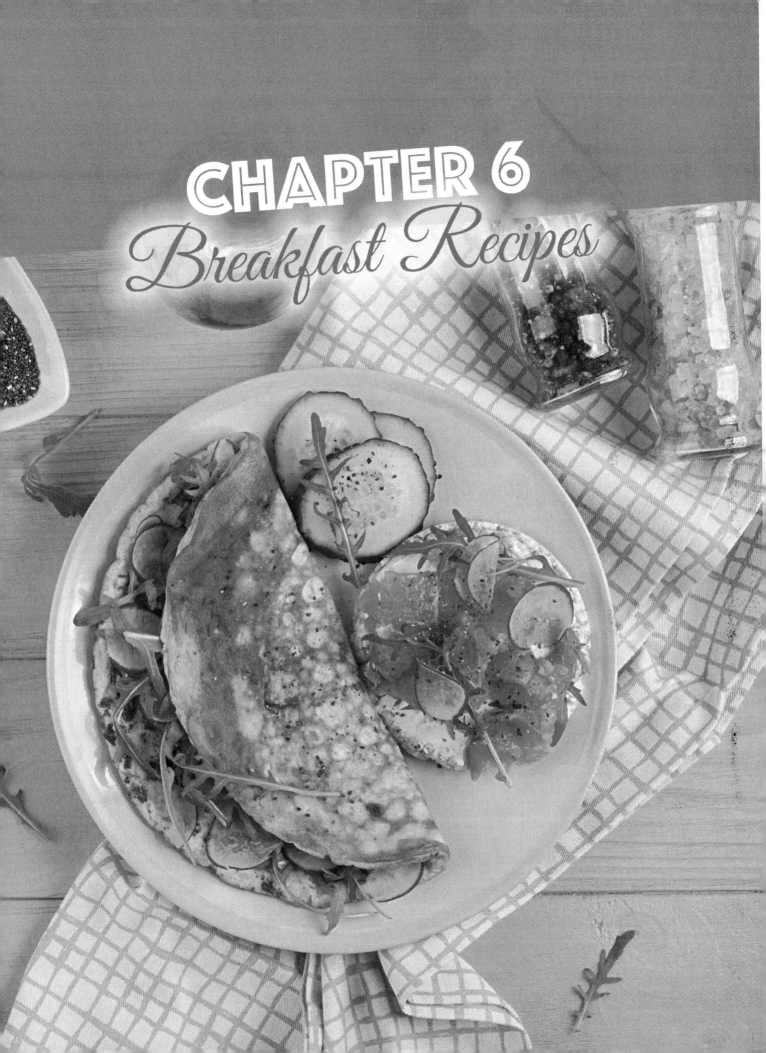

CHAPTER 6
Breakfast Recipes

CHEDDAR & BACON EGG BITES

PREPARATION TIME: 10'   **COOKING TIME:** 8'   **SERVINGS:** 7

1 cup sharp cheddar cheese
1 Tbsp. parsley flakes
4 eggs
4 Tbsp. cream
Hot sauce
1 cup water
½ cup cottage cheese
4 slices bacon

1. Blend the cream, cheddar, cottage, and egg in the blender; 30 seconds. Stir in the parsley. Grease silicone egg bite molds.
2. Divide the crumbled bacon between them. Put the egg batter into each cup.
3. With a piece of foil, cover each mold. Place the trivet with the molds in the pot, then fill with 1 cup water. Steam for 8 minutes.
4. Remove, let rest for 5 minutes.
5. Serve, sprinkled with black pepper and optional hot sauce.

NUTRITION: Calories 443, Fat 8, Fiber 1, Carbs 8, Protein 33

AVOCADO PICO EGG BITES

PREPARATION TIME: 15'   **COOKING TIME:** 10'   **SERVINGS:** 7

Egg bites:
1 cup cottage cheese
½ cup cheese
Mexican blend
¼ cup heavy cream
¼ tsp. chili powder
¼ tsp. cumin
¼ tsp. garlic powder
4 eggs
Pepper
Salt

Pico de Gallo:
1 avocado
1 jalapeno
½ tsp. salt
¼ onion
2 Tbsp. cilantro
2 tsp. lime juice
4 Roma tomatoes

1. Mix all of the Pico de Gallo fixing except for the avocado. Gently fold in the avocado.
2. Blend all the egg bites ingredients in a blender.
3. Spoon 1 tablespoon of Pico de Gallo into each egg bite silicone mold.
4. Place the trivet in the pot then fill with 1 cup water.
5. Put the molds in the trivet. Set to high within 10 minutes. Remove.
6. Serve topped with cheese

NUTRITION: Calories 443, Fat 8, Fiber 1, Carbs 8, Protein 33

SALMON SCRAMBLE

PREPARATION TIME: 10'   COOKING TIME: 5'   SERVINGS: 1

2 smoked salmon pieces
1 organic egg yolk
1/8 tsp. red pepper flakes
Black pepper
2 organic eggs
1 Tbsp. dill
1/8 tsp. garlic powder
1 Tbsp. olive oil

1. Beat all items except salmon and oil. Stir in chopped salmon.
2. Warm-up oil over medium-low heat in a frying pan.
3. Add the egg mixture and cook within 3–5 minutes.
4. Serve.

NUTRITION: Calories 443, Fat 8, Fiber 1, Carbs 8, Protein 33

EGG-CRUST PIZZA

PREPARATION TIME: 5'   COOKING TIME: 15'   SERVINGS: 1-2

¼ tsp. dried oregano, to taste
½ tsp. spike seasoning, to taste
1 ounce mozzarella, chopped into small cubes
6–8 sliced thinly black olives
6 slices turkey pepperoni, sliced into half
4–5 thinly sliced small grape tomatoes
2 eggs, beaten well
1–2 tsp. olive oil

1. Preheat the broiler in an oven, then, in a small bowl, beat well the eggs. Cut the pepperoni and tomatoes into slices, then cut the mozzarella cheese into cubes.
2. Put some olive oil in a skillet over medium heat, then heat the pan for around 1 minute until it begins to get hot. Add in eggs and season with oregano and spike seasoning, then cook for around 2 minutes until the eggs begin to set at the bottom.
3. Drizzle half of the mozzarella, olives, pepperoni, and tomatoes on the eggs, followed by another layer of the remaining half of the above ingredients. Ensure that there is a lot of cheese on the top-most layers. Cover the skillet using a lid and cook until the cheese begins to melt and the eggs are set, for around 3–4 minutes.
4. Place the pan under the preheated broiler and cook until the top has browned and the cheese has melted nicely for around 2–3 minutes. Serve immediately.

NUTRITION: Calories 443, Fat 8, Fiber 1, Carbs 8, Protein 33

BREAKFAST ROLL-UPS

PREPARATION TIME: 5'   COOKING TIME: 15'   SERVINGS: 5 roll-ups

Non-stick cooking spray
5 patties cooked breakfast sausage
5 slices cooked bacon
1/3 cups cheddar cheese, shredded
Pepper and salt
10 large eggs

1. Preheat a skillet on medium to high heat, then, using a whisk, combine together two of the eggs in a mixing bowl.
2. Once the pan is hot, lower the heat to medium-low heat then put in the eggs. If you want to, you can utilize some cooking spray.
3. Season eggs with some pepper and salt.
4. Cover the eggs and leave them to cook for a couple of minutes or until the eggs are almost cooked.
5. Drizzle around 1/3 cup of cheese on top of the eggs, then place a strip of bacon and divide the sausage into two, and place on top.
6. Roll carefully the egg on top of the fillings. The roll-up will almost look like a taquito. If you have a hard time folding over the egg, use a spatula to keep the egg intact until the egg has molded into a roll-up.
7. Put aside the roll-up, then repeat the above steps until you have four more roll-ups; you should have 5 roll-ups in total.

NUTRITION: Calories 443, Fat 8, Fiber 1, Carbs 8, Protein 33

CHORIZO AND MOZZARELLA OMELET

PREPARATION TIME: 4'   COOKING TIME: 60'   SERVINGS: 4

2 eggs
6 basil leaves
2 ounces mozzarella cheese
1 Tbsp. butter
1 Tbsp. water
4 thin slices chorizo
1 tomato, sliced
Salt and black pepper, to taste

1. Whisk the eggs along with the water and some salt and pepper. Melt the butter in a skillet and cook the eggs for 30 seconds.
2. Spread the chorizo slices over. Arrange the tomato and mozzarella over the chorizo. Cook for about 3 minutes. Cover the skillet and cook for 3 minutes, until the omelet is set.
3. When ready, remove the pan from heat; run a spatula around the edges of the omelet and flip it onto a warm plate, folded side down.
4. Serve garnished with basil leaves and green salad.

NUTRITION: Calories 100, Fat 8, Fiber 2, Carbs 8, Protein 2.5

HASHED ZUCCHINI & BACON BREAKFAST

PREPARATION TIME: 5'   **COOKING TIME: 30'**   **SERVINGS: 4**

1 medium zucchini, diced
2 bacon slices
1 egg
1 Tbsp. coconut oil
½ small onion, chopped
1 Tbsp. chopped parsley
¼ tsp. salt

1. Place the bacon in a skillet and cook for a few minutes, until crispy. Remove and set aside.
2. Warm the coconut oil and cook the onion until soft, for about 3-4 minutes, occasionally stirring. Add the zucchini and cook for 10 more minutes, until zucchini is brown and tender, but not mushy. Transfer to a plate and season with salt.
3. Crack the egg into the same skillet and fry over medium heat. Top the zucchini mixture with bacon slices and a fried egg. Serve hot, sprinkled with parsley.

NUTRITION: Calories 100, Fat 8, Fiber 2, Carbs 8, Protein 2.5

YOGURT WAFFLES

PREPARATION TIME: 15'   **COOKING TIME: 25'**   **SERVINGS: 5**

½ cup golden flax seeds meal
½ cup plus 3 tbsp. almond flour
½ Tbsp. granulated erythritol
1 Tbsp. vanilla whey protein powder
¼ tsp. baking soda
½ tsp. organic baking powder
¼ tsp. xanthan gum
Salt
1 large organic egg
1 organic egg
2 Tbsp. unsweetened almond milk
1 ½ Tbsp. unsalted butter
3 oz. plain Greek yogurt

1. Preheat the waffle iron, then grease it.
2. Mix add the flour, erythritol, protein powder, baking soda, baking powder, xanthan gum, and salt.
3. Beat the egg white until stiff peaks. In a third bowl, add 2 egg yolks, whole egg, almond milk, butter, yogurt, and beat.
4. Put egg mixture into the bowl of the flour mixture and mix.
5. Gently fold in the beaten egg whites. Place ¼ cup of the mixture into preheated waffle iron and cook for about 4–5 minutes. Serve.

NUTRITION: Calories 114, Fat 7, Fiber 2, Carbs 11, Protein 28

CHICKEN & ASPARAGUS FRITTATA

PREPARATION TIME: 15'   COOKING TIME: 12   SERVINGS: 4

½ cup grass-fed chicken breast
1/3 cup parmesan cheese
6 organic eggs
Salt
Ground black pepper
1/3 cup boiled asparagus
¼ cup cherry tomatoes
¼ cup mozzarella cheese

1. Warm-up broiler of the oven, then mix parmesan cheese, eggs, salt, and black pepper in a bowl.
2. Melt butter, then cook the chicken and asparagus for 2–3 minutes.
3. Add the egg mixture and tomatoes, and mix. Cook for 4–5 minutes.
4. Remove, then sprinkle with the parmesan cheese.
5. Transfer the wok under the broiler and broil for 3–4 minutes. Slice and serve.

NUTRITION: Calories 114, Fat 7, Fiber 2, Carbs 11, Protein 28

TRADITIONAL SPINACH AND FETA FRITTATA

PREPARATION TIME: 5'   COOKING TIME: 30'   SERVINGS: 4

5 ounces spinach
8 oz. crumbled feta cheese
1-pint halved cherry tomatoes
10 eggs
3 Tbsp. olive oil
4 scallions, diced
Salt and black pepper, to taste

1. Preheat your oven to 350°F.
2. Drizzle the oil in a casserole and place in the oven until heated. In a bowl, whisk the eggs along with the black pepper and salt, until thoroughly combined. Stir in the spinach, feta cheese, and scallions.
3. Pour the mixture into the casserole, top with the cherry tomatoes, and place back in the oven. Bake for 25 minutes until your frittata is set in the middle.
4. When done, remove the casserole from the oven and run a spatula around the edges of the frittata; slide it onto a warm platter. Cut the frittata into wedges and serve with salad.

NUTRITION: Calories 450, Fat 26, Fiber 2, Carbs 4, Protein 6

CAULI FLITTERS

PREPARATION TIME: 10'   **COOKING TIME:** 15'   **SERVINGS:** 2

2 eggs
1 head cauliflower
1 Tbsp. yeast
sea salt, black pepper
1–2 Tbsp. ghee
1 Tbsp. turmeric
2/3 cup almond flour

1. Place the cauliflower into a large pot and start to boil it for 8 mins. Add the florets into a food processor and pulse them.
2. Add the eggs, almond flour, yeast, turmeric, salt, and pepper to a mixing bowl. Stir well. Form into patties.
3. Heat your ghee to medium in a skillet. Form your fritters and cook until golden on each side (3–4 mins).
4. Serve it while hot.

NUTRITION: Calories 450, Fat 26, Fiber 2, Carbs 4, Protein 6

BACON-WRAPPED CHICKEN BREAST

PREPARATION TIME: 10'   **COOKING TIME:** 45'   **SERVINGS:** 4

4 boneless, skinless chicken breast
8 oz. sharp cheddar cheese
8 slices bacon
4 oz. sliced jalapeno peppers
1 tsp garlic powder
Salt and pepper to taste

1. Preheat the oven at around 350°F.
2. Ensure to season both sides of chicken breast well with salt, garlic powder, and pepper. Place the chicken breast on a non-stick baking sheet (foil-covered).
3. Cover the chicken with cheese and add jalapeno slices. Cut the bacon slices in half and then place the four halves over each piece of chicken.
4. Bake for around 30 to 45 minutes at most. If the chicken is set but the bacon still feels undercooked, you may want to put it under the broiler for a few minutes.
5. Once done, serve hot with a side of low-carb garlic parmesan roasted asparagus.

NUTRITION: Calories 605, Fat 23, Fiber 2, Carbs 8, Protein 2

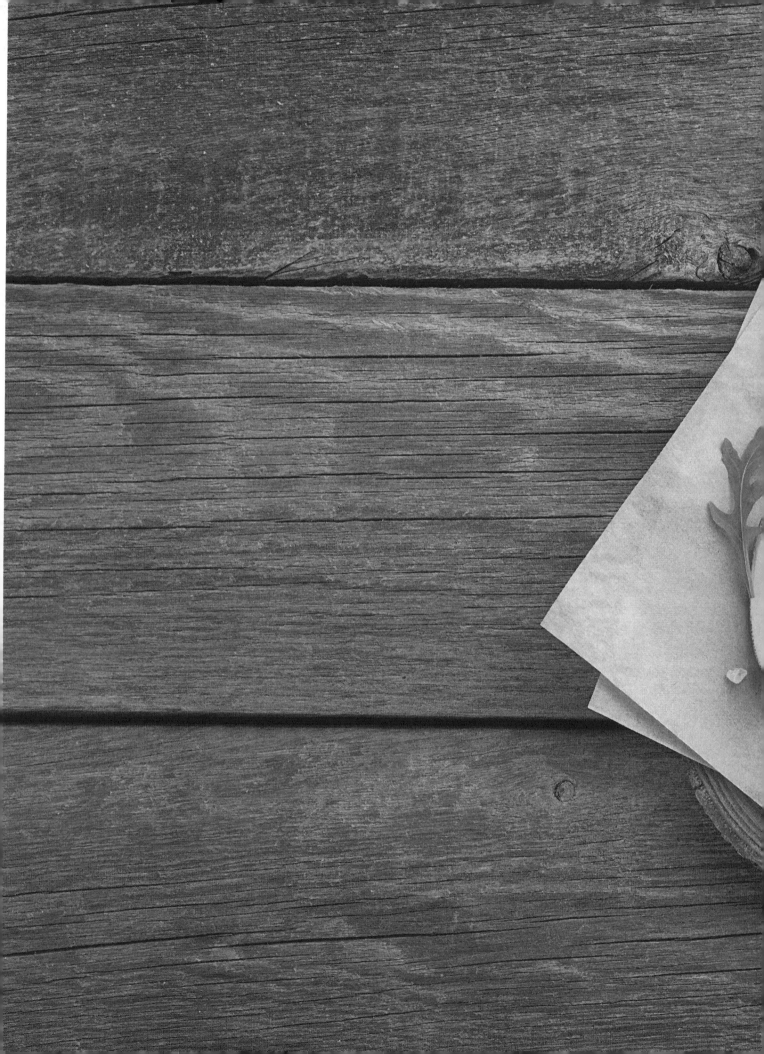

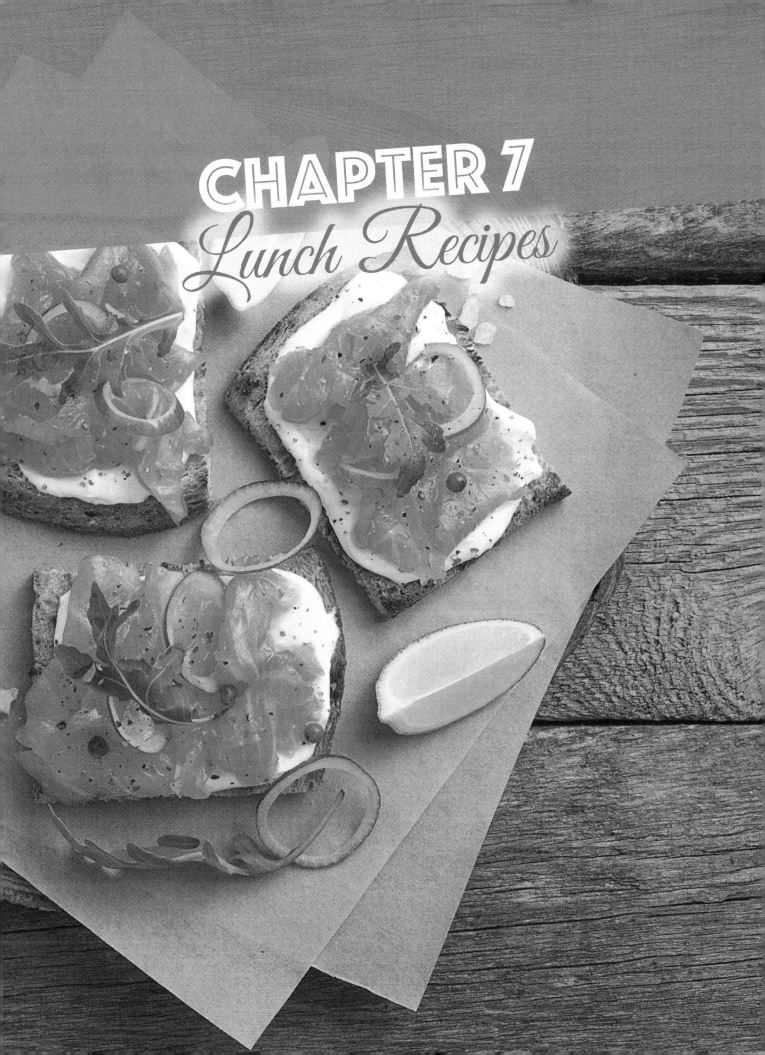

CHAPTER 7
Lunch Recipes

FRESH BROCCOLI AND DILL KETO SALAD

PREPARATION TIME: 15'   **COOKING TIME:** 7   **SERVINGS:** 3

16 oz. broccoli
½ cup mayonnaise
¾ cup chopped dill
Salt
Pepper

1. Boil salted water in a saucepan.
2. Put the chopped broccoli in the pot and boil for 3–5 minutes.
3. Drain and set aside. Once cooled, mix the rest of the fixing.
4. Put pepper and salt, then serve.

NUTRITION: Calories 207, Fat 8, Fiber 2, Carbs 8, Protein 26

LOW-CARB BROCCOLI LEMON PARMESAN SOUP

PREPARATION TIME: 15'   **COOKING TIME:** 15'   **SERVINGS:** 4

3 cups water
1 cup unsweetened almond milk
32 oz. broccoli florets
1 cup heavy whipping cream
¾ cup Parmesan cheese
Salt
Pepper
2 Tbsp. lemon juice

1. Cook broccoli plus water over medium-high heat.
2. Take out 1 cup of the cooking liquid and remove the rest.
3. Blend half the broccoli, reserved cooking liquid, unsweetened almond milk, heavy cream, and salt plus pepper in a blender.
4. Put the blended items to the remaining broccoli and stir with Parmesan cheese and lemon juice.
5. Cook until heated through. Serve with Parmesan cheese on the top.

NUTRITION: Calories 540, Fat 8, Fiber 2, Carbs 8, Protein 6

PROSCIUTTO AND MOZZARELLA BOMB

PREPARATION TIME: 15'   COOKING TIME: 10'   SERVINGS: 4

4 ounces sliced prosciutto
8 ounces mozzarella ball
Olive oil

1. Layer half of the prosciutto vertically. Lay the remaining slices horizontally across the first set of slices. Place mozzarella ball, upside down, onto the crisscrossed prosciutto slices.
2. Wrap the mozzarella ball with the prosciutto slices. Warm up the olive oil in a skillet, crisp the prosciutto, then serve.

NUTRITION: Calories 108, Fat 50, Fiber 2, Carbs 8, Protein 48

GARLIC CHICKEN

PREPARATION TIME: 15'   COOKING TIME: 40'   SERVINGS: 4

2 oz. butter
2 lb. chicken drumsticks
Pepper
Salt
Lemon juice
2 Tbsps. olive oil
7 cloves garlic
½ cup parsley

1. Warmup oven to 250°C.
2. Put the chicken in a baking dish. Add pepper and salt.
3. Add olive oil with lemon juice over the chicken. Sprinkle parsley and garlic on top.
4. Bake within 40 minutes. Serve.

NUTRITION: Calories 200, Fat 8, Fiber 2, Carbs 8, Protein 6

SALMON SKEWERS WRAPPED WITH PROSCIUTTO

PREPARATION TIME: 15'   COOKING TIME: 4'   SERVINGS: 4

¼ cup basil
1 lb. salmon
1 pinch black pepper
4 oz. prosciutto
1 Tbsp. olive oil
8 skewers

1. Start by soaking the skewers in a bowl of water.
2. Cut the salmon fillets lengthwise. Thread the salmon using skewers.
3. Coat the skewers in pepper and basil. Wrap the slices of prosciutto around the salmon.
4. Warm-up oil in a grill pan. Grill the skewers within 4 minutes. Serve.

NUTRITION: Calories 450, Fat 8, Fiber 2, Carbs 8, Protein 24

TURKEY AND CREAM CHEESE SAUCE

PREPARATION TIME: 15'   COOKING TIME: 25'   SERVINGS: 5

2 tbsps. butter
2 lb. turkey breast
2 cups whipping cream
7 oz. cream cheese
1 tbsp. tamari soy sauce
Pepper
Salt
1 ½ oz. capers

1. Warm up the oven at 170°C, then dissolve half butter in an iron skillet.
2. Rub the breast of the turkey with pepper and salt. Fry for 5 minutes.
3. Bake for 10 minutes.
4. Add the drippings of turkey in a pan, cream cheese, and whipping cream. Simmer. Put pepper, soy sauce, and salt. Sauté the small capers in remaining butter.
5. Slice and serve with fried capers and cream cheese sauce.

NUTRITION: Calories 450, Fat 8, Fiber 2, Carbs 8, Protein 24

BUFFALO DRUMSTICKS AND CHILI AIOLI

PREPARATION TIME: 15'   COOKING TIME: 40   SERVINGS: 4

For the chili aioli:
½ cup mayonnaise
1 Tbsp. smoked paprika powder
1 clove garlic

For the chicken:
2 lb. chicken drumsticks
2 Tbsp. each:
White wine vinegar
Olive oil
1 Tbsp. tomato paste

1 tsp. each:
Salt
Paprika powder
Tabasco

1. Warm-up oven to 200°C.
2. Combine the listed marinade fixing. Marinate the chicken drumsticks for 10 minutes.
3. Arrange the chicken drumsticks in the tray. Bake for 40 minutes.
4. Combine the listed items for the chili aioli in a bowl. Serve.

NUTRITION: Calories 263, Fat 8, Fiber 2, Carbs 8, Protein 11

SLOW COOKED ROASTED PORK AND CREAMY GRAVY

PREPARATION TIME: 15'   COOKING TIME: 8 h 15'   SERVINGS: 6

For the creamy gravy:
2 cups whipping cream
Roast juice.

For the pork:
2 lb. pork roast
½ Tbsp. salts
1 bay leaf
5 black peppercorns
3 cups water
2 tsp. thyme
2 cloves garlic
2 oz. ginger

1 Tbsp. each:
Paprika powder
Olive oil
1/3 tsp. black pepper.

1. Warm-up your oven at 100°C.
2. Add the meat, salt, water to a baking dish. Put peppercorns, thyme, and bay leaf. Put in the oven for 8 hours. Remove. Reserve the juices. Adjust to 200°C.
3. Put ginger, garlic, pepper, herbs, and oil. Rub the herb mixture on the meat. Roast the pork for 15 minutes.
4. Slice the roasted meat. Strain the meat juices in a bowl. Boil for reducing it by half.
5. Add the cream. Simmer for 20 minutes. Serve with creamy gravy.

NUTRITION: Calories 263, Fat 8, Fiber 2, Carbs 8, Protein 11

BEEF & VEGGIE CASSEROLE

PREPARATION TIME: 20'   COOKING TIME: 55'   SERVINGS: 6

3 Tbsp butter
1 lb. grass-fed ground beef
1 yellow onion
2 garlic cloves
1 cup pumpkin
1 cup broccoli
2 cups cheddar cheese
1 Tbsp Dijon mustard
6 organic eggs
½ cup heavy whipping cream
Salt
Ground black pepper

1. Cook the beef for 8–10 minutes. Set aside.
2. Cook the onion and garlic for 10 minutes. Add the pumpkin and cook for 5–6 minutes.
3. Add the broccoli and cook for 3–4 minutes. Transfer to the cooked beef, combine.
4. Warm-up oven to 350°F.
5. Put 2/3 of cheese and mustard in the beef mixture, combine.
6. In another mixing bowl, add cream, eggs, salt, and black pepper, and beat.
7. In a baking dish, place the beef mixture and top with egg mixture, plus the remaining cheese.
8. Bake for 25 minutes. Serve.

NUTRITION: Calories 104, Fat 8, Fiber 2, Carbs 8, Protein 2.5

BEEF WITH BELL PEPPERS

PREPARATION TIME: 15'   COOKING TIME: 10'   SERVINGS: 4

1 Tbsp. olive oil
1 lb. grass-fed flank steak
1 red bell pepper
1 green bell pepper
1 Tbsp. ginger
3 Tbsp. low-sodium soy sauce
1 ½ Tbsp. balsamic vinegar
2 tsp. Sriracha

1. Sear the steak slices for 2 minutes. Cook bell peppers for 2–3 minutes.
2. Transfer the beef mixture. Boil the remaining fixing for 1 minute. Add the beef mixture and cook for 1–2 minutes. Serve.

NUTRITION: Calories 443, Fat 8, Fiber 1, Carbs 8, Protein 33

BRAISED LAMB SHANKS

PREPARATION TIME: 15'   **COOKING TIME: 2 h 35'**   **SERVINGS: 4**

4 grass-fed lamb shanks
2 Tbsp. butter
Salt
Ground black pepper
6 garlic cloves
6 rosemary sprigs
1 cup chicken broth

1. Warm-up oven to 450°F.
2. Coat the shanks with butter and put salt plus pepper. Roast for 20 minutes.
3. Remove then reduce to 325°F.
4. Place the garlic cloves and rosemary over and around the lamb.
5. Roast for 2 hours. Put the broth into a roasting pan.
6. Increase to 400°F. Roast for 15 minutes more. Serve.

NUTRITION: Calories 443, Fat 8, Fiber 1, Carbs 8, Protein 33

SHRIMP & BELL PEPPER STIR-FRY

PREPARATION TIME: 20'   **COOKING TIME: 10'**   **SERVINGS: 6**

½ cup low-sodium soy sauce
2 Tbsp. balsamic vinegar
2 Tbsp. Erythritol
1 Tbsp. arrowroot starch
1 Tbsp. ginger
½ tsp. red pepper flakes
3 Tbsp. olive oil
½ red bell pepper
½ yellow bell pepper
½ green bell pepper
1 onion
1 red chili
1½ pounds shrimp
2 scallion greens

1. Mix soy sauce, vinegar, erythritol, arrowroot starch, ginger, and red pepper flakes. Set aside.
2. Stir-fry the bell peppers, onion, and red chili for 1–2 minutes.
3. In the center of the wok, place the shrimp and cook for 1–2 minutes.
4. Stir the shrimp with bell pepper mixture and cook for 2 minutes.
5. Stir in the sauce and cook for 2–3 minutes.
6. Stir in the scallion greens and remove. Serve hot.

NUTRITION: Calories 443, Fat 8, Fiber 1, Carbs 8, Protein 33

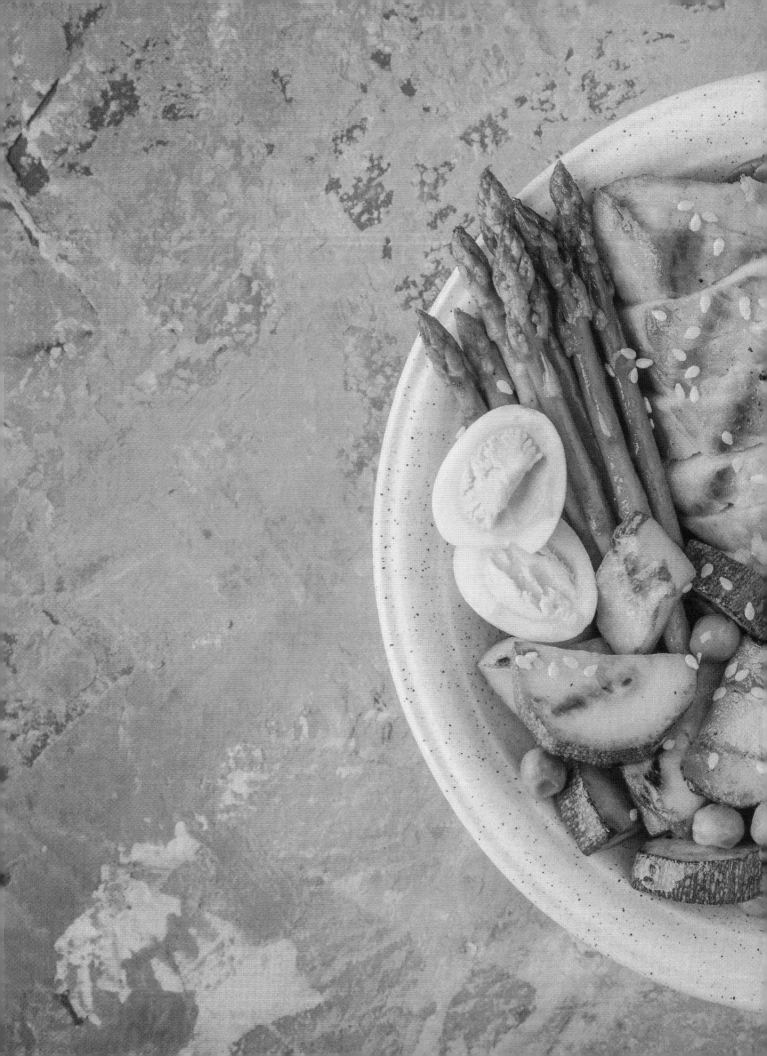

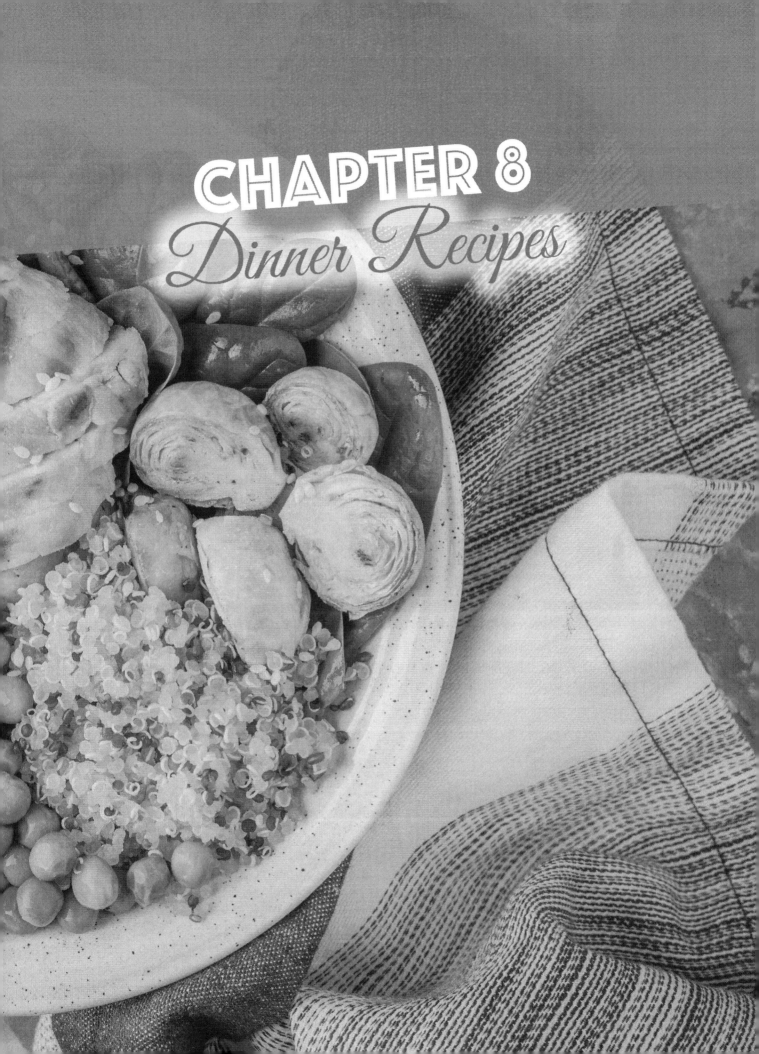

CHAPTER 8
Dinner Recipes

APPLE AND PECANS BOWLS

PREPARATION TIME: 10'   COOKING TIME: 0'   SERVINGS: 4

4 big apples, cored, peeled, and cubed
2 tsp. lemon juice
¼ cup pecans, chopped

1. In a bowl, mix apples with lemon juice and pecans; toss, divide into small bowls, and serve as a snack.

NUTRITION: Calories 233, Fat 8, Fiber 2, Carbs 8, Protein 13

SHRIMP MUFFINS

PREPARATION TIME: 10'   COOKING TIME: 45'   SERVINGS: 6

1 spaghetti squash, peeled and halved
2 Tbsp. avocado mayonnaise
1 cup low-fat mozzarella cheese, shredded
8 oz. shrimp, peeled, cooked, and chopped
1 ½ cups almond flour
1 tsp. parsley, dried
1 garlic clove, minced
Black pepper to the taste
Cooking spray

1. Arrange the squash on a lined baking sheet, introduce in the oven at 375°F, bake for 30 minutes
2. Scrape flesh into a bowl, add pepper, parsley flakes, flour, shrimp, mayo, and mozzarella, and stir well
3. Divide this mixture into a muffin tray greased with cooking spray
4. Bake in the oven at 375°F for 15 minutes and serve them cold as a snack.

NUTRITION: Calories 140, Fat 2, Fiber 4, Carbs 14, Protein 12

ZUCCHINI BOWLS

PREPARATION TIME: 10'   COOKING TIME: 20'   SERVINGS: 12

Cooking spray
½ cup dill, chopped
1 egg
½ cup whole wheat flour
Black pepper, to taste
1 yellow onion, chopped
2 garlic cloves, minced
3 zucchinis, grated

1. In a bowl, mix zucchinis with garlic, onion, flour, pepper, egg, and dill, stir well
2. Shape small bowls out of this mix, arrange them on a lined baking sheet
3. Grease them with some cooking spray, bake at 400°F for 20 minutes, flipping them halfway, divide them into bowls and serve as a snack.

NUTRITION: Calories 120, Fat 1, Fiber 4, Carbs 12, Protein 6

CHEESY MUSHROOMS CAPS

PREPARATION TIME: 10'   COOKING TIME: 30'   SERVINGS: 20

20 white mushroom caps
1 garlic clove, minced
3 Tbsp. parsley, chopped
2 yellow onions, chopped
Black pepper, to taste
½ cup low-fat parmesan, grated
¼ cup low-fat mozzarella, grated
A drizzle olive oil
2 Tbsp. non-fat yogurt

1. Heat up a pan with some oil over medium heat, add garlic and onion, stir, cook for 10 minutes and transfer to a bowl.
2. Add black pepper, garlic, parsley, mozzarella, parmesan, and yogurt, stir well
3. Stuff the mushroom caps with this mix, arrange them on a lined baking sheet
4. Bake in the oven at 400°F for 20 minutes and serve them as an appetizer.

NUTRITION: Calories 120, Fat 1, Fiber 3, Carbs 11, Protein 7

BAKED LEMON & PEPPER CHICKEN

PREPARATION TIME: 20'   COOKING TIME: 25'   SERVINGS: 4

4 chicken breast fillets
Salt, to taste
1 Tbsp. olive oil
1 lemon, sliced thinly
1 Tbsp. maple syrup
2 Tbsp. lemon juice
2 Tbsp. butter
Pepper, to taste

1. Preheat your oven to 425°F.
2. Season chicken with salt.
3. Pour oil into a pan over medium heat.
4. Cook chicken for 5 minutes per side.
5. Transfer chicken to a baking pan.
6. Surround the chicken with lemon slices.
7. Bake in the oven for 10 minutes.
8. Pour in maple syrup and lemon juice into the pan.
9. Put the butter on top of the chicken.
10. Sprinkle with pepper.
11. Bake for another 5 minutes.

NUTRITION: Calories 233, Fat 8, Fiber 2, Carbs 8, Protein 13

SKILLET CHICKEN WITH WHITE WINE SAUCE

PREPARATION TIME: 5'   COOKING TIME: 30'   SERVINGS: 4

4 boneless chicken thighs
1 tsp. garlic powder
1 tsp. dried thyme
1 Tbsp. olive oil
1 Tbsp. butter
1 yellow onion, diced
3 garlic cloves, minced
1 cup dry white wine
½ cup heavy cream
Fresh chopped parsley
Salt and pepper

1. Heat your oil in a skillet. Season your chicken, add it to the skillet, and then cook it for about 5–7 mins.
2. Flip the chicken and cook until looking golden brown.
3. Remove the chicken to a plate.
4. Add butter to the skillet. Then add onions and cook them until softened.
5. Stir in garlic, salt, and pepper, add wine, and cook for 4–5 mins.
6. Stir in the thyme and the heavy cream.
7. Place the breasts back to the skillet and leave to simmer for 2–3 mins. Top them with the parsley.

NUTRITION: Calories: 276, Fats: 21, Carbs: 6, Protein: 25

STIR FRY KIMCHI AND PORK BELLY

PREPARATION TIME: 10'   COOKING TIME: 18'   SERVINGS: 3

300 g pork belly
1 lb. kimchi
1 Tbsp. soy sauce
1 Tbsp. rice wine
1 Tbsp. sesame seeds
1 stalk green onion

1. Slice the pork as thin as possible and marinate it in soy sauce and rice wine for 8–10 mins.
2. Heat a pan. When very hot, add the pork belly and stir-fry until brown.
3. Add the kimchi to the pan and stir-fry for 2 mins to let the flavors completely mix.
4. Turn off the heat and slice the green onion. Top with sesame seeds.

NUTRITION: Calories: 790, Fats: 68, Carbs: 7, Protein: 14

BAKED PESTO CHICKEN

PREPARATION TIME: 5'   COOKING TIME: 35'   SERVINGS: 4

4 chicken breasts (about 1 ½ lb.)
3 Tbsp. basil pesto
8 oz. mozzarella
½ tsp. salt
¼ tsp. black pepper

1. Preheat oven to 350°F.
2. Cover cooking pan with cooking spray. Put the chicken in the base in a single layer and sprinkle with salt and pepper.
3. Spread the pesto on the chicken. Put the mozzarella on top.
4. Heat for 35–45 minutes, until the cheddar is bubbly.
5. Serve.

NUTRITION: Calories 233, Fat 8, Fiber 2, Carbs 8, Protein 13

LOW-CARB PORK MEDALLIONS

PREPARATION TIME: 15'   COOKING TIME: 20'   SERVINGS: 2

1 lb. pork tenderloin
3 medium shallots
¼ cup oil

1. Cut the meat into half-inch-thick slices.
2. Cleave the shallots and put them on a plate.
3. Warm the oil in a skillet.
4. Press each piece of pork into the shallots on both sides. The shallots will stick to the pork if you press firmly.
5. Put the meat slices, coated with shallots, into the warm oil and cook till carried out. Some of the shallots will burn during cooking, but they'll give a heavenly taste to the red meat.
6. Simply cook the beef until it's cooked through.
7. Serve with vegetables.

NUTRITION: Calories 233, Fat 8, Fiber 2, Carbs 8, Protein 13

KETO ROSEMARY ROAST BEEF AND WHITE RADISHES

PREPARATION TIME: 10'   COOKING TIME: 60'   SERVINGS: 8

3 lb. boneless beef roast
2 white daikon radishes
3 Tbsp. rosemary
2 Tbsp. salt, to taste
2 Tbsp. olive oil

1. Preheat oven to 400°F.
2. Spread olive oil, rosemary, and salt over the beef.
3. Put the stripped and severed radishes at the base of a warming dish.
4. Put the beef on the radishes and bake for 1 hour.
5. When done, wrap the burger in foil and let rest for 20 minutes before serving.

NUTRITION: Calories 280, Fat 8, Fiber 3, Carbs 8, Protein 6

BACON-WRAPPED PORK CHOPS

PREPARATION TIME: 10'   COOKING TIME: 30'   SERVINGS: 4

12 oz. bacon package
6–8 boneless pork chops
Salt and pepper

1. Preheat your oven to 350°F.
2. On a plate or cutting board, layout the pork chops.
3. Wrap each piece of pork in uncooked bacon cuts.
4. Place each bacon-wrapped pork chop onto the baking sheet.
5. Crush extra pepper over the highest point of the now bacon-wrapped pork.
6. Cook them for 30 minutes, flipping them at the 15-minute imprint. Serve promptly and enjoy!

NUTRITION: Calories 280, Fat 8, Fiber 3, Carbs 8, Protein 6

LEMON BUTTER SAUCE WITH FISH

PREPARATION TIME: 10'   COOKING TIME: 10'   SERVINGS: 2

150 g thin white fish fillets
4 Tbsps. butter
2 Tbsps. white flour
2 Tbsps. olive oil
1 Tbsp. fresh lemon juice
Salt and pepper
Chopped parsley

1. Place the butter in a small skillet over medium heat. Melt it and leave it, just stirring it casually. After 3 mins, pour into a small bowl.
2. Add lemon juice and season it, set it aside.
3. Dry the fish with paper towels, season it to taste, and sprinkle it with flour.
4. Heat oil in a skillet over high heat. When shimmering, add the fish and cook around 2–3 mins.
5. Remove to a plate and serve with the sauce. Top with parsley.

NUTRITION: Calories: 371, Fats: 27, Carbs: 3, Protein: 30

PRESSURE COOKER CRACK CHICKEN

PREPARATION TIME: 5'   COOKING TIME: 25'   SERVINGS: 8

2 lbs. boneless chicken thighs.
2 slices bacon
8 oz. cream cheese
1 scallion sliced
½ cup shredded cheddar
1 ½ tsp. garlic and onion powder
1 tsp. red pepper flakes and dried dill
Salt and pepper
2 Tbsp. apple cider vinegar
1 Ttbsp. dried chives

1. On the pressure cooker, use sauté mode and wait for it to heat up. Add the bacon and cook until crispy. Then set aside on a plate.
2. Add everything in the pot, except the cheddar cheese. On Manual high, pressure-cook them for 15 mins, and then take them out.
3. On a large plate, shred the chicken and then return to the pot and add the cheddar.
4. Top with the bacon and scallion.

NUTRITION: Calories: 437, Fats: 28, Carbs: 5, Protein: 41

SPINACH STUFFED CHICKEN BREASTS

PREPARATION TIME: 25'   COOKING TIME: 15'   SERVINGS: 4

1 ½ lb. chicken breasts
4 ozs. cream cheese
¼ cup frozen spinach
½ cup mozzarella
4 oz. artichoke hearts
¼ cup Greek yogurt
Salt and pepper
2 Tbsp. olive oil

1. Pound the breasts about 1 inch thick. Cut each chicken down the middle but don't cut through it. Make a pocket for the filling.
2. In a bowl, combine the Greek yogurt, mozzarella, cream cheese, artichoke, and spinach. Next, season it. Mix until well-combined.
3. Fill all breasts equally with your mixture.
4. In a skillet over medium heat, add the oil and place your chicken. Cover the skillet and cook for 5–6 mins, turning the heat up in the last 1-2 mins.

NUTRITION: Calories: 288, Fats: 18, Carbs: 3, Protein: 31

CHAPTER 9
Meat Recipes

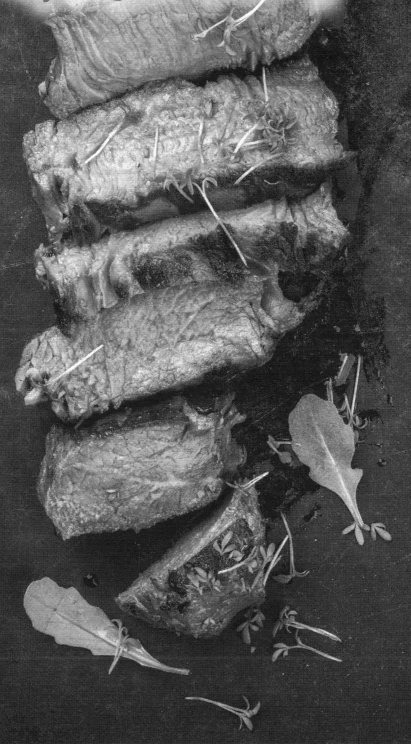

BEEF TACO BAKE

PREPARATION TIME: 15'   COOKING TIME: 1 h   SERVINGS: 6

For Crust:
3 organic eggs
4 oz. cream cheese
½ tsp. taco seasoning
1/3 cup heavy cream
8 oz. cheddar cheese

For Topping:
1 lb. grass-fed ground beef
4 oz. green chilies
¼ cup sugar-free tomato sauce
3 tsp. taco seasoning
8 ounces cheddar cheese

1. Warm-up oven to 375°F.
2. For the crust: beat the eggs, and cream cheese, taco seasoning, and heavy cream.
3. Place cheddar cheese in the baking dish. Spread cream cheese mixture over cheese.
4. Bake for 25-30 minutes. Remove then set aside within 5 minutes.

For topping:
5. Cook the beef for 8–10 minutes.
6. Stir in the green chilies, tomato sauce, and taco seasoning and transfer.
7. Place the beef mixture over the crust and sprinkle with cheese. Bake for 18-20 minutes.
8. Remove, then slice and serve.

NUTRITION: Calories: 569, Carbs: 3.8, Fiber: 0.2, Protein: 38.7

SPICY CITRUS MEATBALLS

PREPARATION TIME: 5'   COOKING TIME: 8 h   SERVINGS: 6

1 ½ lb. ground beef
1 egg
1 Tbsp. Worcestershire sauce
1 Tbsp. garlic chili sauce
½ cup onion, diced
1 cup zucchini, shredded
2 Tbsp. olive oil
3 cups green beans, trimmed
1 cup beef stock
1 Tbsp. crushed red pepper flakes
¼ cup soy sauce
1 tsp. orange extract
1 tsp. black pepper

1. In a bowl, combine the ground beef, egg, Worcestershire sauce, garlic chili sauce, onion and zucchini. Mix well.
2. Take the spoonful of the meat mixture and form them into golf ball-sized meatballs.
3. Pour the olive oil into a skillet over medium heat.
4. Place the meatballs in the skillet and cook just until browned on all sides.
5. Place the green beans in the slow cooker.
6. Transfer the meatballs from the skillet to the slow cooker.
7. Combine the beef stock, crushed red pepper flakes, soy sauce, orange extract, and black pepper. Mix well and pour into the slow cooker.
8. Cover and cook on low for 8 hours.

NUTRITION: Calories 120, Fat 8, Fiber 2, Carbs 12, Protein 33

BEEF IN SAUCE

PREPARATION TIME: 10'   **COOKING TIME: 9 h**   **SERVINGS: 4**

1 lb. beef stew meat, chopped
1 tsp. gram masala
1 cup water
1 Tbsp. flour
1 tsp. garlic powder
1 onion, diced

1. Whisk flour with water until smooth and pour the liquid into the slow cooker.
2. Add gram masala and beef stew meat.
3. After this, add onion and garlic powder.
4. Close the lid and cook the meat on low for 9 hours.
5. Serve the cooked beef with thick gravy from the slow cooker.

NUTRITION: Calories 120, Fat 8, Fiber 2, Carbs 12, Protein 33

BEEF WITH GREENS

PREPARATION TIME: 15'   **COOKING TIME: 8 h**   **SERVINGS: 3**

1 cup fresh spinach, chopped
9 oz. beef stew meat, cubed
1 cup Swiss chard, chopped
2 cups water
1 tsp. olive oil
1 tsp. dried rosemary

1. Heat olive oil in the skillet.
2. Add beef and roast it for 1 minute per side.
3. Then transfer the meat into the slow cooker.
4. Add Swiss chard, spinach, water, and rosemary.
5. Close the lid and cook the meal on Low for 8 hours.

NUTRITION: Calories 210, Fat 12, Fiber 2, Carbs 8, Protein 26

BEEF AND SCALLIONS BOWL

PREPARATION TIME: 10'   COOKING TIME: 5 h   SERVINGS: 4

1 lb. beef stew meat, cubed
1 tsp. chili powder
2 oz. scallions, chopped
1 cup corn kernels, frozen
1 cup water
2 Tbsp. tomato paste
1 tsp. minced garlic

1. Mix water with tomato paste and pour the liquid into the slow cooker.
2. Add chili powder, beef, corn kernels, and minced garlic.
3. Close the lid and cook the meal on high for 5 hours.
4. When the meal is cooked, transfer the mixture to the bowls and top with scallions.

NUTRITION: calories 291, fat 9, fiber 2, carbs 8, protein 20

MEATBALLS IN CHEESE SAUCE

PREPARATION TIME: 20'   COOKING TIME: 25'   SERVINGS: 5

For Meatballs:
1 lb. ground pork
1 organic egg
2 oz. Parmesan cheese
½ Tbsp. dried basil
1 tsp. garlic powder
½ tsp. onion powder
Salt
ground black pepper
3 Tbsp. olive oil
For Sauce:
1 can sugar-free tomatoes
2 Tbsp. butter
7 oz. spinach
2 Tbsp. parsley
5 oz. mozzarella cheese
Salt
Ground black pepper

For meatballs:
1. Mix all the fixing except oil in a large bowl. Make small-sized balls from the mixture.
2. Cook the meatballs for 3–5 minutes. Add the tomatoes. Simmer for 15 minutes.
3. Stir fry the spinach for 1–2 minutes in butter. Put salt and black pepper.
4. Remove then put the cooked spinach, parsley, and mozzarella cheese into meatballs and stir.
5. Cook for 1–2 minutes. Remove and serve.

NUTRITION: Calories 170, Fat 8, Fiber 2, Carbs 8, Protein 4

CHOCOLATE CHILI

PREPARATION TIME: 15'   COOKING TIME: 2 h 15'   SERVINGS: 8

2 Tbsp. olive oil
1 small onion
1 green bell pepper
4 garlic cloves
1 jalapeño pepper
1 tsp. dried thyme
2 Tbsp. red chili powder
1 Tbsp. ground cumin
2 lb. lean ground pork
2 cups fresh tomatoes
4 oz. sugar-free tomato paste
1 ½ Tbsp. cacao powder
2 cups chicken broth
1 cup water
Salt
Ground black pepper
¼ cup cheddar cheese

1. Sauté the onion and bell pepper for 5–7 minutes.
2. Add the garlic, jalapeño pepper, thyme, and spices, and sauté for 1 minute.
3. Add the pork and cook for 4–5 minutes. Stir in the tomatoes, tomato paste, and cacao powder and cook for 2 minutes.
4. Add the broth and water, boil. Simmer, covered for 2 hours. Stir in the salt and black pepper. Remove then top with cheddar cheese and serve.

NUTRITION: Calories 100, Fat 8, Fiber 2, Carbs 12, Protein 19

BEEF & CABBAGE STEW

PREPARATION TIME: 15'   COOKING TIME: 2 h 10'   SERVINGS: 4

2 lb. grass-fed beef stew meat
1 1/3 cups hot chicken broth
2 yellow onions
2 bay leaves
1 tsp Greek seasoning
Salt
Ground black pepper
3 celery stalks
1 package cabbage
1 can sugar-free tomato sauce
1 can sugar-free whole plum tomatoes

1. Sear the beef for 4–5 minutes. Stir in the broth, onion, bay leaves, Greek seasoning, salt, and black pepper, and boil. Adjust the heat to low and cook for 1¼ hours.
2. Stir in the celery and cabbage and cook for 30 minutes. Stir in the tomato sauce and chopped plum tomatoes and cook, uncovered for 15–20 minutes. Stir in the salt, discard bay leaves and serve.

NUTRITION: Calories 150, Fat 7, Fiber 2, Carbs 8, Protein 10

BEEF & MUSHROOM CHILI

PREPARATION TIME: 15'   COOKING TIME: 3 h 10'   SERVINGS: 8

2 lb. grass-fed ground beef
1 yellow onion
½ cup green bell pepper
½ cup carrot
4 oz. mushrooms
2 garlic cloves
1 can sugar-free tomato paste
2 Tbsp. red chili powder
1 Tbsp. ground cumin
1 tsp. ground cinnamon
1 tsp. red pepper flakes
½ tsp. ground allspice
Salt
Ground black pepper
4 cups water
½ cup sour cream

1. Cook the beef for 8–10 minutes. Stir in the remaining fixing except for sour cream and boil.
2. Cook on low, covered, for 3 hours.
3. Top with sour cream and serve.

NUTRITION: Calories 150, Fat 7, Fiber 2, Carbs 8, Protein 10

STEAK WITH CHEESE SAUCE

PREPARATION TIME: 15'   COOKING TIME: 17'   SERVINGS: 4

18 oz. grass-fed filet mignon
Salt
Ground black pepper
2 Tbsp. butter
½ cup yellow onion
5 ¼ oz. blue cheese
1 cup heavy cream
1 garlic clove
Ground nutmeg

1. Cook onion for 5-8 minutes. Add the blue cheese, heavy cream, garlic, nutmeg, salt, and black pepper, and stir.
2. Cook for about 3-5 minutes.
3. Put salt and black pepper in filet mignon steaks. Cook the steaks for 4 minutes per side.
4. Transfer and set aside.
5. Top with cheese sauce, then serve.

NUTRITION: Calories 178, Fat 8, Fiber 2, Carbs 8, Protein 36

STEAK WITH BLUEBERRY SAUCE

PREPARATION TIME: 15'   COOKING TIME: 20'   SERVINGS: 4

For Sauce:
2 Tbsp. butter
2 Tbsp. yellow onion
2 garlic cloves
1 tsp. thyme
1 1/3 cups beef broth
2 Tbsp. lemon juice
¾ cup blueberries

For Steak:
2 Tbsp. butter
4 grass-fed flank steaks
Salt
Ground black pepper

For the sauce:
1. sauté the onion for 2–3 minutes.
2. Add the garlic and thyme and sauté for 1 minute. Stir in the broth and simmer for 10 minutes.

For the steak:
3. Put salt and black pepper.
4. Cook steaks for 3–4 minutes per side.
5. Transfer and put aside. Add sauce in the skillet and stir. Stir in the lemon juice, blueberries, salt, and black pepper, and cook for 1-2 minutes. Put blueberry sauce over the steaks.
6. Serve.

NUTRITION: Calories 233, Fat 8, Fiber 2, Carbs 8, Protein 13

GRILLED STEAK

PREPARATION TIME: 15'   COOKING TIME: 12   SERVINGS: 6

1 tsp. lemon zest
1 garlic clove
1 Tbsp. red chili powder
1 Tbsp. paprika
1 Tbsp. ground coffee
Salt
Ground black pepper
2 grass-fed skirt steaks

1. Mix all the ingredients except steaks.
2. Marinate the steaks and keep them aside for 30–40 minutes.
3. Grill the steaks for 5–6 minutes per side.
4. Remove then cool before slicing. Serve.

NUTRITION: Calories 233, Fat 8, Fiber 2, Carbs 8, Protein 13

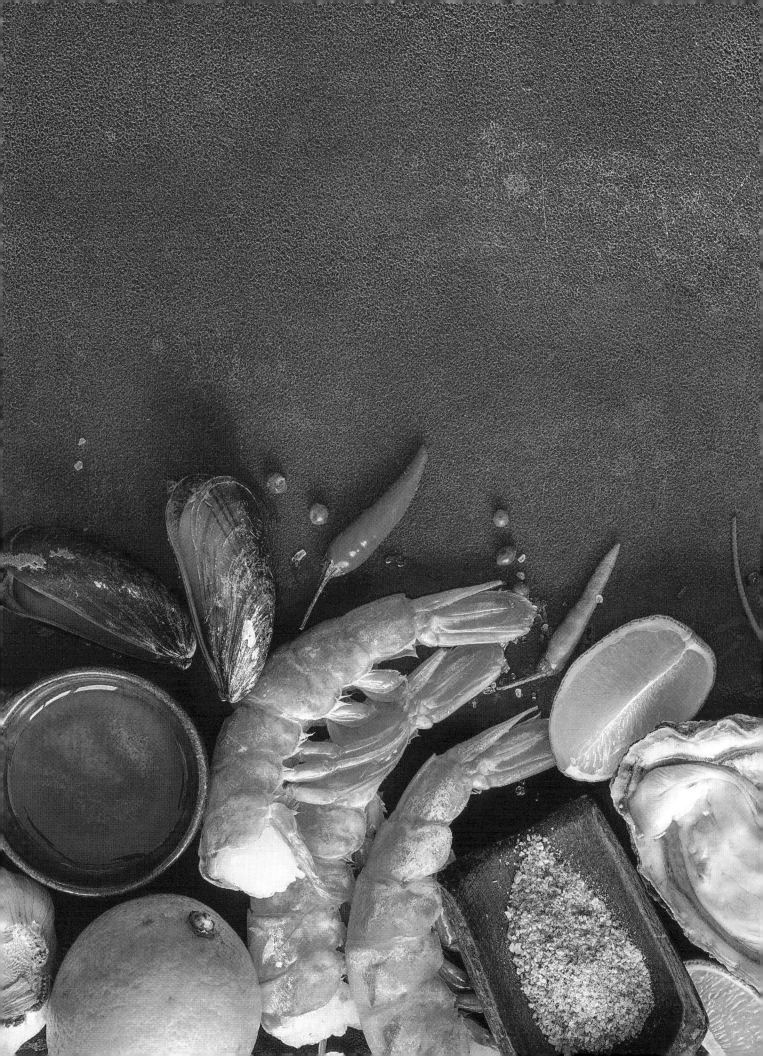

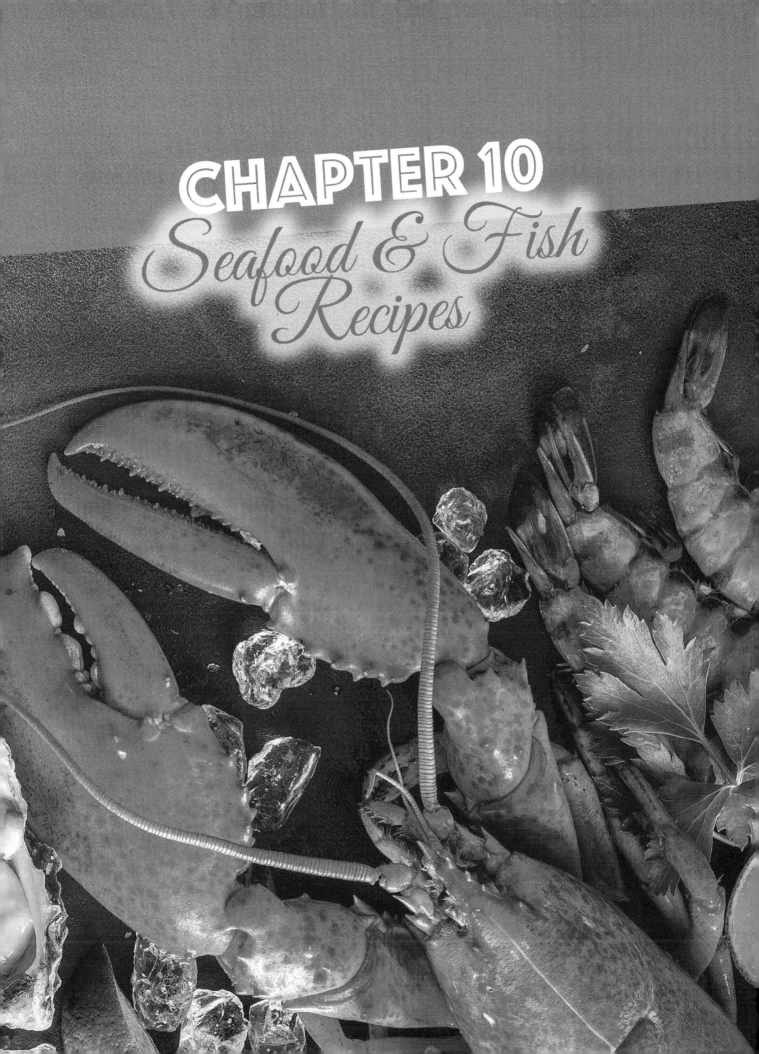

CHAPTER 10
Seafood & Fish Recipes

CREAMY TUNA, SPINACH, AND EGGS PLATES

PREPARATION TIME: 5'   COOKING TIME: 0'   SERVINGS: 2

2 oz. spinach leaves
2 oz. tuna, packed in water
2 eggs, boiled
4 Tbsp. cream cheese, full-fat

Seasoning:
¼ tsp. salt
1/8 tsp. ground black pepper

1. Take two plates and evenly distribute spinach and tuna between them.
2. Peel the eggs, cut them into half, and divide them between the plates, and then season with salt and black pepper.
3. Serve with cream cheese.

NUTRITION: 212 Calories; 14.1 Fats; 18 Protein; 1.9 Net Carb; 1.3 Fiber;

BAKED FISH FILLETS WITH VEGETABLES IN FOIL

PREPARATION TIME: 15'   COOKING TIME: 40'   SERVINGS: 3

1 lb. cod
1 red bell pepper
6 cherry tomatoes
1 leek
¼ onion
½ zucchini
1 clove garlic
2 Tbsp. olives
1 oz. butter
2 Tbsp. olive oil
½ lemon sliced
Coriander leaves
Salt
Pepper

1. Warm-up the oven to 400°F. Transfer all the vegetables to a baking sheet lined with foil.
2. Cut the fish into bite-sized and add to the vegetables. Add salt and pepper, olive oil, and add pieces of butter. Bake for 35–40 minutes. Serve.

NUTRITION: Calories 240, Fat 8, Fiber 2, Carbs 8, Protein 27

SHRIMP CREOLE

PREPARATION TIME: **10'** COOKING TIME: **4 h** SERVINGS: **6**

1 cup onion
1 garlic clove
1 cup red bell pepper
1 cup celery
1 tsp. salt
1/4 tsp. pepper
6 drops Tabasco
½ tsp. Creole seasoning
4 oz. canned tomato sauce
14 oz. canned whole tomatoes
2 lb. shrimp
½ cup white rice

1. Add all the ingredients to the slow cooker, except for the shrimp.
2. Cook on High for 4 hours.
3. In the last 30 minutes of your cooking, add the shrimp.

NUTRITION: Calories 240, Fat 8, Fiber 2, Carbs 8, Protein 27

SALMON AND SCALLOPED POTATOES

PREPARATION TIME: **10'** COOKING TIME: **60'** SERVINGS: **4**

Cooking spray
3 Tbsp. flour
Salt and pepper
16 oz. salmon
5 potatoes
½ cup onion
¼ cup water
10 oz. cream mushroom soup
Pinch nutmeg

1. Grease your slow cooker with cooking spray.
2. Sprinkle with a little bit of flour.
3. Sprinkle with salt and pepper.
4. Arrange a layer of half of the salmon flakes, half of the potatoes, and half of the chopped onions.
5. Make another set of layers.
6. Mix the water and soup.
7. Pour into the slow cooker. Add the nutmeg.
8. Cover the pot. Cook on low for 9 hours.

NUTRITION: Calories 290, Fat 4, Fiber 2, Carbs 8, Protein 25

TILAPIA IN LEMON PEPPER SAUCE

PREPARATION TIME: 10'   **COOKING TIME: 60'**   **SERVINGS: 4**

4 fillets tilapia
16 spears asparagus
8 Tbsp. freshly squeezed lemon juice
8 Tbsp. pepper
2 Tbsp. butter

1. Cut the foil.
2. Put each tilapia fillet into the foil.
3. Place 4 spears of asparagus on each tilapia.
4. Sprinkle each fillet with ¼ tsp. pepper.
5. Sprinkle 2 tbsp. lemon juice onto each fillet.
6. Add ½ tbsp. butter on each fillet.
7. Wrap the fillet with the foil.
8. Place wrapped tilapia in the slow cooker.
9. Cook on High for 2 hours.

NUTRITION: Calories 290, Fat 4, Fiber 2, Carbs 8, Protein 25

ASIAN STYLE SALMON

PREPARATION TIME: 10'   **COOKING TIME: 10'**   **SERVINGS: 4**

16 oz. frozen veggies
Salt and pepper
10 oz. salmon fillets
2 Tbsp. lemon juice
2 Tbsp. soy sauce
2 Tbsp. honey
1 tsp. sesame honey
1 tsp. sesame seeds

1. Put the vegetables on a slow cooker.
2. Rub the salt and pepper onto the salmon fillets.
3. Put the salmon fillets on top of the vegetables.
4. Combine the lemon juice, soy sauce, and honey.
5. Pour this mixture over the salmon.
6. Sprinkle with sesame seeds.
7. Set cooker to low. Cook for 3 hours.

NUTRITION: Calories 265, Fat 8, Fiber 2, Carbs 8, Protein 36

BAKED SALMON WITH ALMONDS AND CREAM SAUCE

PREPARATION TIME: 10'   COOKING TIME: 20'   SERVINGS: 2

Almond Crumbs Creamy Sauce:
3 Tbsp. almonds
2 Tbsp. almond milk
½ cup cream cheese
Salt

Fish:
1 salmon fillet
1 tsp. coconut oil
1 Tbsp. lemon zest
1 tsp. salt
White pepper

1. Cut the salmon in half. Rub the salmon with lemon zest, salt, and pepper. Marinade for 20 minutes.
2. Fry the fish on both sides. Top with almond crumbs and bake for 10 to 15 minutes.
3. Remove and put aside.
4. Place the baking dish on fire and add the cream cheese. Combine the fish baking juices and the cheese. Mix, then pour the sauce onto the fish. Serve.

NUTRITION: Calories 265, Fat 8, Fiber 2, Carbs 8, Protein 36

SHRIMP AND SAUSAGE BAKE

PREPARATION TIME: 15'   COOKING TIME: 20'   SERVINGS: 4

2 Tbsp. olive oil
6 oz. chorizo sausage
½ lb. shrimp
½ small sweet onion
1 tsp. garlic
¼ cup Herbed Chicken Stock
Pinch red pepper flakes
1 red bell pepper

1. Sauté the sausage for 6 minutes. Add the shrimp and sauté for 4 minutes. Remove both and set aside.
2. Cook the red pepper, onion, and garlic in the skillet for 4 minutes.
3. Put the chicken stock along with the cooked sausage and shrimp. Simmer for 3 minutes.
4. Stir in the red pepper flake and serve.

NUTRITION: Calories 120, Fat 8, Fiber 2, Carbs 12, Protein 33

TUNA AND AVOCADO

PREPARATION TIME: 5'   COOKING TIME: 0'   SERVINGS: 2

2 oz. tuna, packed in water
1 avocado, pitted
8 green olives
½ cup mayonnaise, full-fat

Seasoning:
1/3 tsp. salt
¼ tsp. ground black pepper

1. Cut avocado into half, then remove the pit, scoop out the flesh and distribute between two plates.
2. Add tuna and green olives and then season with salt and black pepper.
3. Serve with mayonnaise.

NUTRITION: 680 Calories; 65.6 Fats; 10.2 Protein; 2.2 Net Carb; 9.7 Fiber

GARLIC OREGANO FISH

PREPARATION TIME: 5'   COOKING TIME: 12'   SERVINGS: 2

2 pacific whitening fillets
1 tsp. minced garlic
1 Tbsp. butter, unsalted
2 tsp. dried oregano

Seasoning:
1/3 tsp. salt
¼ tsp. ground black pepper

1. Turn on the oven, then set it to 400°F and let it preheat.
2. Meanwhile, take a small saucepan, place it over low heat, add butter and when it melts, stir in garlic and cook for 1 minute, remove the pan from heat.
3. Season fillets with salt and black pepper, and place them on a baking dish greased with oil.
4. Pour butter mixture over fillets, then sprinkle with oregano and bake for 10 to 12 minutes until thoroughly cooked.
5. Serve.

NUTRITION: 199.5 Calories; 7 Fats; 33.5 Protein; 0.9 Net Carb; 0.1 Fiber

BACON-WRAPPED SALMON

PREPARATION TIME: 5'   COOKING TIME: 10'   SERVINGS: 2

2 salmon fillets, cut into four pieces
4 slices bacon
2 tsp. avocado oil
2 Tbsp. mayonnaise

Seasoning:
½ tsp. salt
½ tsp. ground black pepper

1. Turn on the oven, then set it to 375°F and let it preheat.
2. Meanwhile, place a skillet pan, place it over medium-high heat, add oil and let it heat.
3. Season salmon fillets with salt and black pepper, wrap each salmon fillet with a bacon slice, then add to the pan and cook for 4 minutes, turning halfway through.
4. Then transfer skillet pan containing salmon into the oven and cook salmon for 5 minutes until thoroughly cooked.
5. Serve salmon with mayonnaise

NUTRITION: 190.7 Calories; 16.5 Fats; 10.5 Protein; 0 Net Carb; 0 Fiber

FISH AND EGG PLATE

PREPARATION TIME: 5'   COOKING TIME: 10'   SERVINGS: 2

2 eggs
1 Tbsp. butter, unsalted
2 pacific whitening fillets
½ oz. chopped lettuce
1 scallion, chopped
Seasoning:
3 Tbsp. avocado oil
1/3 tsp. salt
1/3 tsp. ground black pepper

1. Cook the eggs, and for this, take a frying pan, place it over medium heat, add butter and when it melts, crack the egg in the pan and cook for 2 to 3 minutes until fried to desired liking.
2. Transfer the fried egg to a plate and then cook the remaining eggs in the same manner.
3. Meanwhile, season fish fillets with ¼ tsp each of salt and black pepper.
4. When eggs have fried, sprinkle salt and black pepper on them, then add 1 tbsp. oil into the frying pan, add fillets, and cook for 4 minutes per side until thoroughly cooked.
5. When done, distribute fillets to the plate, add lettuce and scallion, drizzle with remaining oil, and then serve.

NUTRITION: Calories 120, Fat 8, Fiber 2, Carbs 12, Protein 33

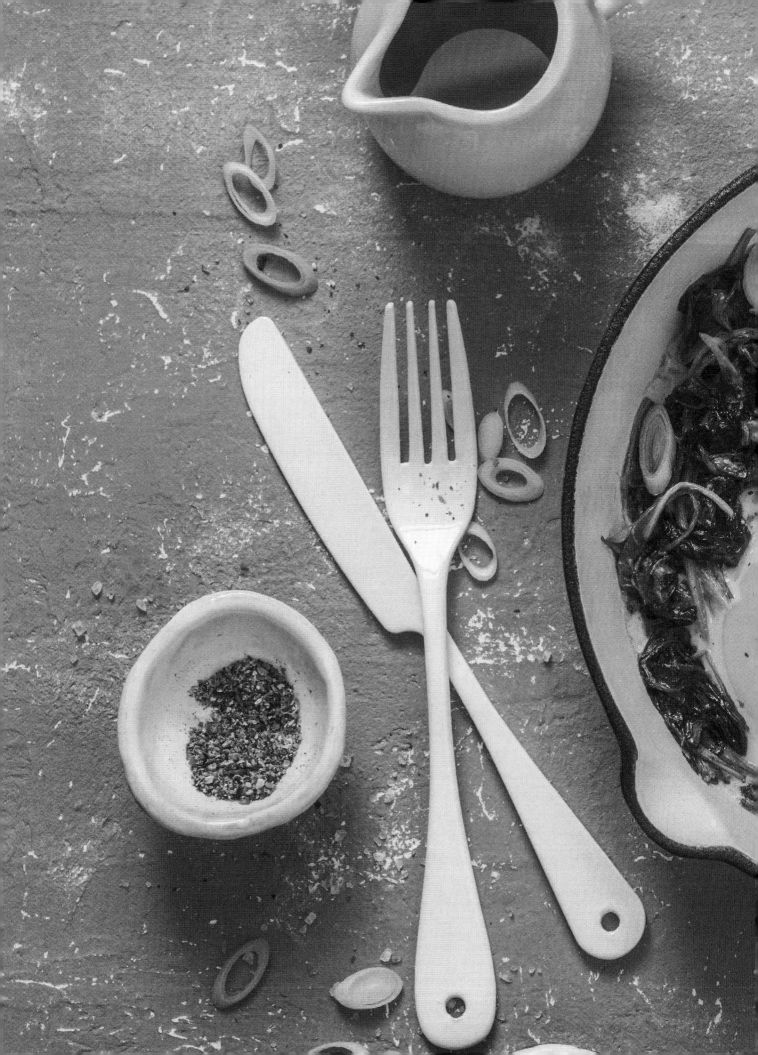

CHAPTER 11
Vegetarian & Vegan Recipes

BOK CHOY STIR FRY WITH FRIED BACON SLICES

PREPARATION TIME: 17'   COOKING TIME: 15'   SERVINGS: 2

2 cup Bok choy; chopped
2 Garlic cloves; minced
2 Bacon slices; chopped
A drizzle avocado oil
Salt and black pepper, to taste.

1. Take a pan and heat it with oil over medium heat.
2. When the oil is hot, add bacon and keep stirring it until it's brown and crispy.
3. Transfer them to paper towels to drain out the excess oil.
4. Now, bring the pan to medium heat, and in it add garlic and bok choy.
5. Again, stir it and cook it for 5 minutes.
6. Now, drizzle and add some salt, pepper, and fried bacon, and stir them for another 1 minute.
7. Turn off the heat and divide them into plates to serve.

NUTRITION: Calories: 50; Fat: 1; Fiber: 1; Carbs: 2; Protein: 2

BACON AVOCADO BOMBS

PREPARATION TIME: 10'   COOKING TIME: 10'   SERVINGS: 2

1 avocado, halved, pitted
4 slices bacon
2 Tbsp. grated parmesan cheese

1. Turn on the oven and broiler, and let it preheat.
2. Meanwhile, prepare the avocado, and for that, cut it in half, then remove its pit, and then peel the skin.
3. Evenly one-half of the avocado with cheese, replace with the other half of avocado and then wrap avocado with bacon slices.
4. Take a baking sheet, line it with aluminum foil, place wrapped avocado on it, and broil for 5 minutes per side, flipping carefully with tong halfway.
5. When done, cut each avocado in half crosswise and serve

NUTRITION: 378 Calories; 33.6 Fats; 15.1 Protein; 0.5 Net Carb; 2.3 Fiber

EGG IN A HOLE WITH EGGPLANT

PREPARATION TIME: 5'   COOKING TIME: 15'   SERVINGS: 2

1 large eggplant
2 eggs
1 Tbsp. coconut oil, melted
1 tsp. unsalted butter
2 Tbsp. chopped green onions

Seasoning:
¾ tsp. ground black pepper
¾ tsp. salt

1. Set the grill and let it preheat at the high setting.
2. Meanwhile, prepare the eggplant, and for this, cut two slices from eggplant, about 1-inch thick, and reserve the remaining eggplant for later use.
3. Brush slices of eggplant with oil, season with salt on both sides, then place the slices on the grill and cook for 3 to 4 minutes per side.
4. Transfer grilled eggplant to a cutting board, let it cool for 5 minutes and then make a hole in the center of each slice by using a cookie cutter.
5. Take a frying pan, place it over medium heat, add butter and when it melts, add eggplant slices in it and crack an egg into each hole.
6. Let the eggs cook for 3 to 4 minutes, then carefully flip the eggplant slice and continue cooking for 3 minutes until the egg has thoroughly cooked.
7. Season egg with salt and black pepper, transfer them to a plate, then garnish with green onions and serve.

NUTRITION: 184 Calories; 14.1 Fats; 7.8 Protein; 3 Net Carb; 3.5 Fiber

BROCCOLI-CAULIFLOWER STEW

PREPARATION TIME: 25'   COOKING TIME: 15'   SERVINGS: 5

2 Bacon slices, chopped
1 Cauliflower head, separated into florets
1 Broccoli head, separated into florets
2 tbsp. Butter
2 Garlic cloves, minced

1. Put a pan on medium heat and dissolve the butter and the garlic. Add the bacon slices to brown for 3 minutes all over.
2. Mix in broccoli and cauliflower florets to cook for 2 minutes.
3. Pour water over it and cover with the lid and let cook for 10 minutes.
4. Season with pepper and salt and puree soup with a dipping blend.
5. Let boil slowly for some minutes on medium heat.
6. Serve into bowls.

NUTRITION: Calories- 128, Carbs- 4, Protein- 6, Fiber- 7, Fats- 2

BOK CHOY MUSHROOM SOUP

PREPARATION TIME: 25' **COOKING TIME:** 15' **SERVINGS:** 4

2 Bacon strips, chopped
3 cups Beef stock
1 bunch Bok choy, chopped
1 Onion, chopped
3 Tbsp. Parmesan cheese, grated
3 Tbsp. Coconut aminos
2 Tbsp. Worcestershire sauce
½ Tbsp. Red pepper flakes
1 ½ cups Mushrooms, chopped
Black Pepper
Salt

1. Put bacon in a saucepan over medium-high heat to brown until crispy, then take to paper towels to drain.
2. To medium heat, add the mushrooms and onions to the pan and cook for 15 minutes.
3. Pour in the stock, pepper flakes, aminos, bok choy, Worcestershire sauce, salt and pepper, and mix.
4. Cook until bok choy is tender.
5. Serve into bowls and sprinkle with Parmesan cheese and bacon.

NUTRITION: Calories- 100, Carbs- 1, Protein- 5, Fiber- 9, Fats- 5

TASTY RADISH SOUP

PREPARATION TIME: 30' **COOKING TIME:** 45' **SERVINGS:** 4

1 Chopped onion
Salt
2 Chopped celery stalk
6 cup Chicken stock
3 Tbsps. Coconut oil
2 bunches Quartered radishes
Black pepper
6 Minced garlic cloves

1. Set the pan over medium heat and preheat the oil
2. Stir in the celery, onion, and garlic to cook until soft, about 5 minutes
3. Stir in the stock, radishes, and seasonings.
4. Cover and simmer to boil for 15 minutes
5. Enjoy while still hot

NUTRITION: Calories: 131, Fat: 12, Fiber: 8, Carbs: 4, Protein: 1

BELL PEPPER EGGS

PREPARATION TIME: 10' **COOKING TIME: 4'** **SERVINGS: 2**

1 green bell pepper,
2 eggs

Seasoning:
1 tsp. coconut oil
¼ tsp. salt
¼ tsp. ground black pepper

1. Prepare pepper rings, and for this, cut out two slices from the pepper, about ¼-inch, and reserve the remaining bell pepper for later use.
2. Take a skillet pan, place it over medium heat, grease it with oil, place pepper rings in it, and then crack an egg into each ring.
3. Season eggs with salt and black pepper, cook for 4 minutes or until eggs have cooked to the desired level.
4. Transfer eggs to a plate and serve.

NUTRITION: 110.5 Calories; 8 Fats; 7.2 Protein; 1.7 Net Carb; 1.1 Fiber

FRITTATA WITH SPINACH AND MEAT

PREPARATION TIME: 10' **COOKING TIME: 20'** **SERVINGS: 2**

4 oz. ground turkey
3 oz. spinach leaves
1/3 tsp. minced garlic
1/3 tsp. coconut oil
2 eggs

Seasoning:
1/3 tsp. salt
¼ tsp. ground black pepper

1. Turn on the oven, then set it to 400°F, and let it preheat.
2. Meanwhile, take a skillet pan, place it over medium heat, and add spinach and cook for 3 to 5 minutes until spinach leaves have wilted, remove the pan from heat.
3. Take a small heatproof skillet pan, place it over medium heat, add ground turkey and cook for 5 minutes until thoroughly cooked.
4. Then add spinach, season with salt and black pepper, stir well, then remove the pan from heat and spread the mixture evenly in the pan.
5. Crack eggs in a bowl, season with salt and black pepper, then pour this mixture over spinach mixture in the pan and bake for 10 to 15 minutes until frittata has thoroughly cooked and the top is golden brown.
6. When done, let frittata rest in the pan for 5 minutes, then cut it into slices and serve.

NUTRITION: 166 Calories; 13 Fats; 10 Protein; 0.5 Net Carb; 0.5 Fiber

AVOCADO EGG BOAT WITH CHEDDAR

PREPARATION TIME: 5'   COOKING TIME: 15'   SERVINGS: 2

1 avocado, halved, pitted
2 eggs
2 Tbsp. chopped bacon
2 Tbsp. shredded cheddar cheese

Seasoning:
1/8 tsp. salt
1/8 tsp. ground black pepper

1. Turn on the oven, then set it to 400°F and let it preheat.
2. Meanwhile, prepare avocado, and for this, cut it into half lengthwise, and then remove the pit.
3. Scoop out some of the flesh from the center, crack an egg into each half, and then sprinkle with bacon and season with salt and black pepper.
4. Sprinkle cheese over egg and avocado, and then bake for 10 to 15 minutes or until the yolk has cooked to the desired level.
5. Serve.

NUTRITION: 263.5 Calories; 21.4 Fats; 12 Protein; 1.3 Net Carb; 4.6 Fiber

FRIED GARLICKY BACON AND BOK CHOY BROTH

PREPARATION TIME: 17'   COOKING TIME: 15'   SERVINGS: 2

2 cups Bok choy, chopped
A drizzle avocado oil
2 Bacon slices, chopped
2 Garlic cloves, minced
Black pepper
Salt

1. Put bacon in a pan on medium heat and let crisp. Remove and let drain on paper towels.
2. Add bok choy and garlic to the pan and let cook for 4 minutes.
3. Season with pepper and salt and put the bacon back into the pan.
4. Let cook for 1 minute and serve.

NUTRITION: Calories- 116, Carbs- 8, Protein- 3, Fiber- 8, Fats- 1

NUTRITIONAL MUSTARD GREENS AND SPINACH SOUP

PREPARATION TIME: 25'   **COOKING TIME:** 15'   **SERVINGS:** 6

5 cup Spinach; torn
½ tsp. Fenugreek seeds
1 tsp. Cumin seeds
1 Tbsp. Jalapeno;
      chopped
5 cup Mustard greens;
      chopped
2 tsp. Ghee -
½ tsp. Paprika
1 Tbsp. Avocado oil
1 tsp. Coriander seeds
1 cup Yellow onion;
      chopped
1 Tbsp. Garlic; minced
1 Tbsp. Ginger; grated
½ tsp. Turmeric;
      ground
3 cup Coconut milk
Salt and black pepper, to
      taste.

1. Add coriander, fenugreek, and cumin seed in a heated pot with oil over medium-high heat.
2. Now, stir and brow them for 2 minutes.
3. In the same pot, add onions and again stir them for 3 minutes.
4. Now, after the onion's cooked, add half of the garlic, jalapenos, ginger, and turmeric.
5. Again, give it a good stir and cook for another 3 minutes.
6. Add some more mustard greens, spinach and saute everything for 10 minutes.
7. After it's done, add milk, salt, pepper before blending the soup with an immersion blender.
8. Now take another pan and heat it up over medium heat with some ghee drizzled on it.
9. In it, add garlic, paprika, and give it a good stir before turning off the heat.
10. Bring the soup to heat over medium heat and transfer them into soup bowls.
11. Top it with some drizzles of ghee and paprika. Now it's ready to serve hot.

NUTRITION: Calories: 143; Fat: 6; Fiber: 3; Carbs: 7; Protein: 7

BAKED RADISHES

PREPARATION TIME: 30'   **COOKING TIME:** 35'   **SERVINGS:** 4

1 Tbsp. Chopped chives,
15 Sliced radishes,
Salt
Vegetable oil cooking spray
Black pepper

1. Line your baking sheet well, then spray with the cooking spray
2. Set the sliced radishes on the baking tray, then sprinkle with cooking oil
3. Add the seasonings, then top with chives
4. Set the oven for 10 minutes at 375°F, allow to bake
5. Turn the radishes to bake for 10 minutes
6. Serve cold

NUTRITION: Calories: 63, Fat: 8, Fiber: 3, Carbs: 6, Protein: 1

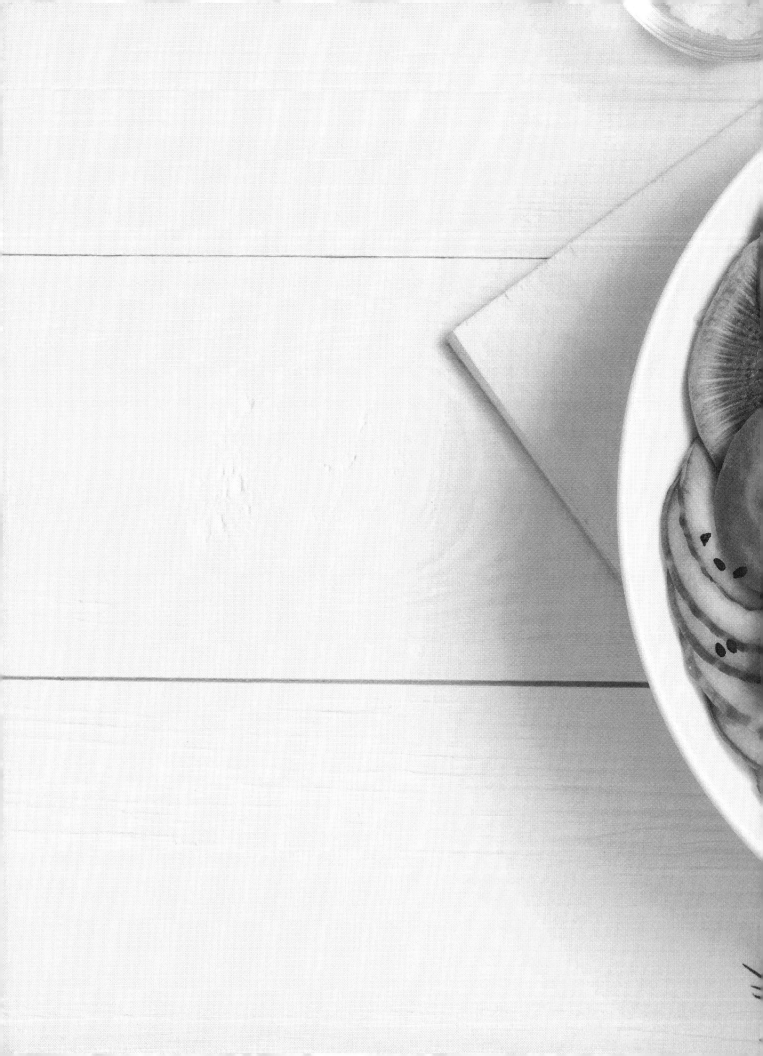

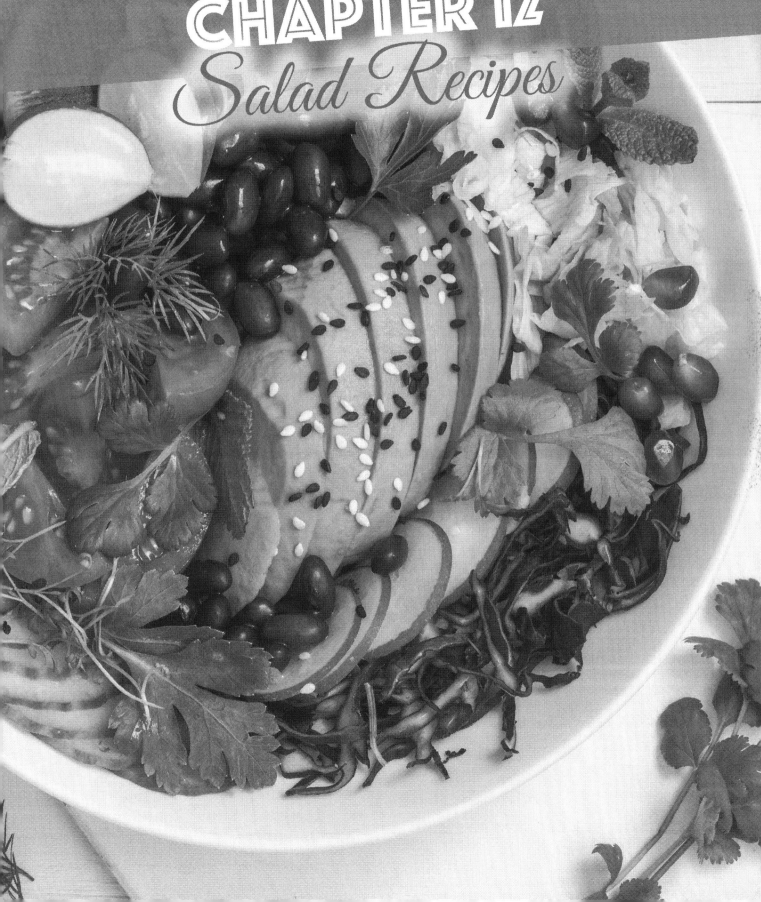

CHAPTER 12
Salad Recipes

KETO CHICKEN BLT SALAD

PREPARATION TIME: 10'   COOKING TIME: 10'   SERVINGS: 4

1 lb. boneless chicken thighs
1 oz. butter
0.5 lb. bacon
4 oz. cherry tomatoes
10 oz. Romaine lettuce
Salt and pepper

Garlic mayonnaise:
0.75 cup mayonnaise
0.5 Tbsp. garlic powder

1. Blend mayonnaise and garlic powder in a little bowl and put in a safe spot.
2. Spare the oil in the skillet. Sear the bacon cuts to spread until crispy. Set aside and keep warm.
3. Shred the chicken and season with salt and pepper. Sear in a similar skillet as the bacon until brilliant darker and completely cooked.
4. Wash and shred the lettuce; make sure to utilize a spotless cutting board and blade (not the same as the one utilized when taking care of the crude chicken). Place the lettuce on a plate and top with chicken, bacon, tomatoes, and a healthy touch of garlic mayonnaise.

NUTRITION: Calories 185, Fat 12, Fiber 2, Carbs 4, Protein 11

KETO TUNA SALAD WITH BOILED EGGS

PREPARATION TIME: 10'   COOKING TIME: 10'   SERVINGS: 2

4 oz. celery stalks
2 scallions
5 oz. tuna in olive oil
0.5 lemon, zest, and juice
0.5 cup mayonnaise
1 tsp. Dijon mustard
4 eggs
6 oz. Romaine lettuce
4 oz. cherry tomatoes
2 tbsp olive oil
Salt and pepper

1. Cut celery and scallions finely. Add to a medium-sized bowl together with fish, lemon, mayonnaise, and mustard. Blend to join, and season with salt and pepper. Put in a safe spot.
2. Add eggs to a sauce container, and include water until it covers the eggs. Heat to the point of boiling and let stew for 5–6 minutes (delicate medium) or 8–10 minutes (hardboiled).
3. Place in super cold water promptly when done to make the eggs simpler to strip. Cut them into wedges or parts.
4. Place fish blend and eggs on a bed of romaine lettuce. Add tomatoes and sprinkle olive oil on top. Season with salt and pepper to taste.

NUTRITION: Calories 280, Fat 8, Fiber 2, Carbs 7, Protein 8

SPICY SHRIMP SALAD

PREPARATION TIME: 10'   COOKING TIME: 10'   SERVINGS: 2

2 avocados
0.5 lime, juice
5 oz. cucumber
2 oz. baby spinach
3 Tbsp. olive oil, for frying
1 garlic clove, pressed
2 tsp. chili powder or sambal oelek
10 oz. shrimp, peeled
Fresh cilantro, for serving
2 Tbsp. hazelnuts or salted peanuts (optional)

Ginger dressing:
0.25 cup light olive oil or avocado oil
1 Tbsp. fresh ginger, minced
0.5 lime, juice
0.5 Tbsp. tamari soy sauce
0.5 garlic clove, pressed
Salt and pepper, to taste

1. Split avocado down the middle and expel pit. Scoop out avocado pieces with a spoon and cut in cuts. Crush some lime juice over avocado. Strip and cut cucumber.
2. Join spinach, avocado, and cucumber on a plate. Season with ocean salt.
3. Sear garlic and bean stew in oil. Include shrimp and broil on each side for a couple of minutes if crude. Pre-cooked shrimp should just be warmed up rapidly. Salt and pepper to taste.
4. Include shrimp on top of vegetables and sprinkle with nuts and cilantro.
5. Blend elements for dressing with an immersion blender and sprinkle over a plate of mixed greens

NUTRITION: Calories 340, Fat 15, Fiber 2, Carbs 18, Protein 30

KETO COBB SALAD WITH RANCH DRESSING

PREPARATION TIME: 10'   COOKING TIME: 10'   SERVINGS: 2

2 eggs
3 oz. bacon
0.5 rotisserie chicken
2 oz. blue cheese
1 avocado
1 tomato
5 oz. iceberg lettuce
1 Tbsp. fresh chives (optional)
Salt and ground black pepper
Easy ranch dressing:
3 Tbsp. mayonnaise
1 Tbsp. ranch seasoning
2 Tbsp. water
Salt and ground black pepper

1. Begin by setting up the dressing. Consolidate mayonnaise, ranch seasoning, and water. Season with salt and pepper, and put in a safe spot.
2. Place the eggs in bubbling water for 8–10 minutes. Cool in ice water for simpler stripping. Hack them generally.
3. Broil bacon in a hot dry skillet until fresh. Cut flame-broiled chicken into little pieces and slash up vegetables. In case you're beginning with raw chicken, sear it in the bacon fat, and season with salt and pepper to taste. Disintegrate the blue cheddar.
4. Convey everything on a bed of shredded or torn lettuce. Season with salt and pepper (particularly the eggs).
5. Shower with dressing and top with finely cleaved chives.

NUTRITION: Calories 200, Fat 8, Fiber 2, Carbs 8, Protein

KETO AVOCADO, BACON, AND GOAT-CHEESE SALAD

PREPARATION TIME: 10'   **COOKING TIME:** 10'   **SERVINGS:** 4

0.5 lemon, the juice
0.5 cup mayonnaise
0.5 cup olive oil
2 Tbsp. heavy whipping cream
8 oz. goat cheese
8 oz. bacon
2 avocados
4 oz. walnuts
4 oz. arugula lettuce

1. Preheat the stove to 400°F (200°C) and place parchment paper in a preparing dish.
2. Cut the goat cheddar into round half-inch (~1 cm) cuts and place in the heating dish. Prepare on the upper rack until brilliant.
3. Broil the bacon in a container until firm.
4. Cut the avocado into pieces and put it over the arugula. Include the seared bacon and goat cheddar. Sprinkle nuts on top.
5. Utilizing an immersion blender, make a plate of mixed greens dressing with the juice from a large portion of a lemon, hand-crafted mayonnaise, olive oil, and maybe several tablespoons of overwhelming whipping cream. Season with salt and pepper to taste.

NUTRITION: Calories 354, Fat 14, Fiber 2, Carbs 16, Protein 26

KETO ASIAN BEEF SALAD

PREPARATION TIME: **10'**   COOKING TIME: **10'**   SERVINGS: **2**

Sesame mayonnaise:
1 cup mayonnaise
1 Tbsp. sesame oil
0.5 Tbsp. lime juice
Salt and pepper
Beef:
1 Tbsp. olive oil
1 Tbsp. fish sauce
1 Tbsp. grated fresh ginger
1 tsp. chili flakes
0.66 lb ribeye steaks
Salad:
3 oz. cherry tomatoes
2 oz. cucumber
3 oz. lettuce
0.5 red onion
Fresh cilantro
1 tsp. sesame seeds
2 scallions

1. Set up the sesame mayonnaise by blending mayo with the sesame oil and lime juice. Season with salt and pepper. Put in a safe spot.
2. Blend all elements for the meat marinade and fill a plastic pack. Include the hamburger and marinate for 15 minutes or more at room temperature.
3. Hack all vegetables for the plate of mixed greens, aside from the scallions, into nibble-measured pieces. Distribute between two plates.
4. Warmth a medium griddle over medium warmth. Add sesame seeds to the dry skillet and toast them for a few minutes, or until they're daintily cooked and fragrant. Put in a safe spot.
5. Pat the meat dry on the two sides with paper towels. On high heat, burn for a minute or two on each side, and afterward diminish warmth to medium-low, cooking until meat is medium, and after that move to a cutting board.
6. Broil the scallions for a moment in a similar container.
7. Cut the meat, over the grain, into dainty cuts. Place meat and scallions over the vegetables.
8. Top with broiled sesame seeds and present with a touch of sesame mayonnaise as an afterthought.

NUTRITION: Calories 320, Fat 8, Fiber 2, Carbs 0, Protein 34

KETO CAULIFLOWER POTATO SALAD

PREPARATION TIME: 10'   COOKING TIME: 10'   SERVINGS: 2

Cauliflower salad:
25 oz. large cauliflower
Salt and ground black pepper
0.5 cup water
5 oz. bacon
3 celery stalks
0.5 red onion
2 Tbsp. fresh chives

Dressing:
1.5 cups mayonnaise
0.75 Tbsp. Dijon mustard
0.75 Tbsp. cider vinegar
1 pinch salt
1 pinch ground black pepper

Cauliflower salad:

1. Preheat the flame broil on low heat.
2. Slash cauliflower into nibble estimated pieces. Gap and spot pieces on two separate sheets of aluminum foil in a level layer. Season with salt and pepper.
3. Lift foil edges so it somewhat covers the cauliflower. Pour 1/4 cup of water onto every cauliflower bundle. Cover with another bit of foil and wrap appropriately, ensure the water doesn't get away. Barbecue for 15–20 minutes as an afterthought, maintaining a strategic distance from the hot focus and leaving space for the bacon.
4. Lay bacon cuts in a flame broil skillet with high edges. Flame broil for 10–15 minutes until firm. Flip them part of the way through.
5. Hack celery stalks into little pieces, finely dice the onion and chives.
6. Remove bacon from the barbecue. Once cooled, cleave into little pieces.
7. Take out cauliflower and cautiously unwrap. Permit to cool totally. Once cooled, include cauliflower in a major bowl. Add bacon, celery, onions, and chives. Spare a couple of pieces for fixing.

Dressing:

8. In a bowl, consolidate mayonnaise, mustard, and juice vinegar. Season with salt and pepper. Blend until joined.
9. Pour over the cauliflower plate of mixed greens and hurl to join equitably. Top with bacon and chives.

NUTRITION: Calories 320, Fat 8, Fiber 2, Carbs 0, Protein 34

ITALIAN MAYONNAISE

PREPARATION TIME: 10'   COOKING TIME: 10'   SERVINGS: 4

1 cup mayonnaise
1 Tbsp. italian seasoning, see ingredients below

Italian seasoning:
3 Tbsp. dried basil
3 Tbsp. dried oregano
3 Tbsp. dried parsley
1 tbsp. garlic powder
1 tsp. onion powder
1 tsp. dried thyme
1 tsp. dried rosemary
1 tsp. dried sage
0.25 tsp. ground black pepper
0.25 tsp. chili flakes
1 Tbsp. sea salt (optional)

1. Blend mayonnaise and Italian flavoring in a little bowl.
2. Put in a safe spot for 30 minutes or more to give the flavors a chance to create. Check if it needs extra flavoring.
3. Keep refrigerated for up to 4–5 days.

Italian seasoning:
4. Altogether combine the flavors. Fill a container with a tight-fitting top.
5. If you utilize entire seeds, crush in a processor either ahead of time or when cooking.
6. Keep the flavors in a dim, dry, and room temperature territory. Little tin jars are incredible.
7. Make a major cluster to keep going for 4–6 months; after this, the flavors will lose some flavor and shading. They won't turn sour yet will be less ground-breaking.

NUTRITION: Calories 282, Fat 4, Fiber 2, Carbs 14, Protein 3

SPINACH SALAD WITH HOT BACON FAT DRESSING

PREPARATION TIME: 10'   COOKING TIME: 10'   SERVINGS: 4

Spinach salad:
6 cup fresh spinach
2 hard-boiled eggs, chopped
2 oz. chopped bacon
0.33 cup parmesan cheese, finely grated (optional)

Hot bacon fat dressing:
0.5 cup bacon fat or light olive oil
0.25 cup apple cider vinegar
1 Tbsp. Dijon mustard
Salt
Ground black pepper

1. Wash the spinach and remove intense closures. Dry the leaves. Distribute the spinach uniformly among four serving of mixed greens plates.
2. Top with hard-bubbled eggs and bacon isolated uniformly among the plates. Sprinkle Parmesan cheddar on top whenever wanted.
3. Utilize a little pot to warm the bacon fat. Add the apple juice vinegar and remaining fixings. Serve warm and blend just before pouring.
4. Dress plate of mixed greens plates with hot bacon fat vinaigrette and serve right away.

NUTRITION: calories 150, fat 8, fiber 22, carbs 8, protein 13

SLOW-COOKED CHICKEN WITH BROCCOLI SALAD

PREPARATION TIME: **10'**   COOKING TIME: **10'**   SERVINGS: **4**

5 lime leaves
1 Tbsp. coriander seed
1 Tbsp. ground ginger
0.5 tsp. ground black pepper
1 cup Greek yogurt or another type
of yogurt with a high-fat content
3 lb. chicken drumsticks
2 tsp. salt
2 limes for serving (optional)

Broccoli Salad:
1 lb broccoli
1 cup mayonnaise
0.5 cup chopped fresh cilantro
Salt and pepper

1. Pound the flavors and blend with the yogurt. Salt the chicken and put it in a plastic sack. Pour in the yogurt marinade and back rub it into the chicken.
2. Marinate (in the icebox) for 2–3 hours or medium-term. On the off chance that you are in a surge, marinate for any event 15 minutes at room temperature.
3. Put chicken and marinade in a moderate cooker and cook on high heat for three hours or low for 6–8 hours. Remove and let cool. You can plan up to this stage multi-day ahead.
4. Set up the barbecue and completion off the chicken with a pleasant caramelized surface, around 5–10 minutes on each side, contingent upon size and warmth.
5. On the off chance that you don't have a flame broil, you can burn the bubbled chicken on the stove utilizing the oven setting. Cut the limes down the middle and sear or barbecue nearby the chicken, chop side down. They add a great flavor.

NUTRITION: Calories 150, Fat 8, Fiber 22, Carbs 8, Protein 13

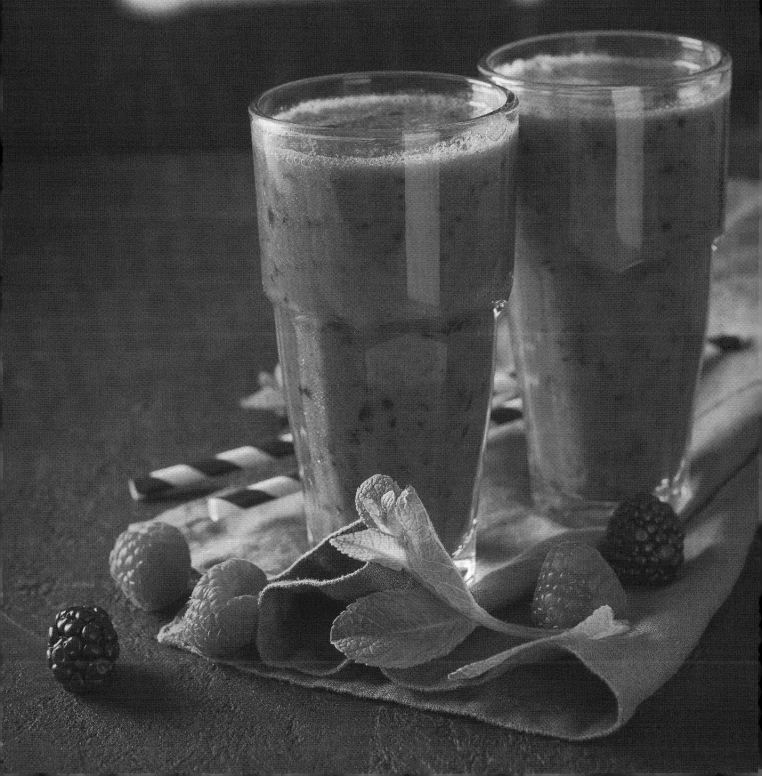

CHAPTER 13
Smoothies Recipes

THE STRAWBERRY ALMOND SMOOTHIE

PREPARATION TIME: 5'   COOKING TIME: 0'   SERVINGS: 1

16 oz. unsweetened almond milk, vanilla
1 pack stevia
4 oz. heavy cream
1 scoop vanilla whey protein
¼ cup frozen strawberries, unsweetened

1. Add all the listed ingredients to a blender.
2. Blend on high until smooth and creamy.
3. Enjoy your smoothie.

NUTRITION: Calories 275, Fat 20, Fiber 2, Carbs 8, Protein 20

EARLY MORNING FRUIT SMOOTHIE

PREPARATION TIME: 5'   COOKING TIME: 0'   SERVINGS: 1

1 cup Spring mix salad blend
2 cup water
3 medium blackberries, whole
1 packet Stevia, optional
1 Tbsp. avocado oil
1 Tbsp. coconut flakes shredded and unsweetened
2 Tbsp. pecans, chopped
1 Tbsp. hemp seed
1 Tbsp. sunflower seed

1. Add all the listed ingredients to a blender.
2. Blend on high until smooth and creamy.
3. Enjoy your smoothie.

NUTRITION: Calories 200, Fat 8, Fiber 2, Carbs 8, Protein 6

CHOCOLATE-FLAVORED CHAI SMOOTHIE

PREPARATION TIME: 5'   COOKING TIME: 0'   SERVINGS: 1

1 ½ cups boiling water
1 black tea bag
¼ tsp. ginger
¼ tsp. cinnamon
¼ tsp. cardamom powder
2 packets Stevia or as desired
½ cup coconut milk
2 Tbsp. Dutch-processed cocoa powder, unsweetened
1 Tbsp. MCT oil

1. In a large mug, mix boiling water, ginger, cinnamon, and cardamom powder. Add the tea bag and let it steep until the liquid is cool. Remove the tea bag and squeeze out excess liquid and discard. Refrigerate liquid with spices until chilled. You can even transfer it to an ice cube tray and freeze it.
2. Add all ingredients to a blender.
3. Blend until smooth and creamy.
4. Serve and enjoy.

NUTRITION: Calories 198, Fat 12, Fiber 2, Carbs 2, Protein 35

RASPBERRY-COFFEE CREAMY SMOOTHIE

PREPARATION TIME: 5'   COOKING TIME: 0'   SERVINGS: 1

½ cup coconut milk
1 ½ cup brewed coffee, chilled
¼ cup Raspberries
¼ avocado fruit
2 packets Stevia or more to taste
1 tsp. chia seeds

1. Add all ingredients to a blender.
2. Blend until smooth and creamy.
3. Serve and enjoy.

NUTRITION: Calories 340, Fat 23, Fiber 2, Carbs 8, Protein 28

BLUEBERRY AND GREENS SMOOTHIE

PREPARATION TIME: 5'   **COOKING TIME:** 0'   **SERVINGS:** 1

½ cup coconut milk
1 ½ cup water
½ cup blueberries
2 packets Stevia, or as needed
1 cup arugula
1 Tbsp. hemp seeds

1. Add all ingredients to a blender.
2. Blend until smooth and creamy.
3. Serve and enjoy.

NUTRITION: Calories 270, Fat 18, Fiber 1, Carbs 3, Protein 22

AVOCADO AND GREENS SMOOTHIE

PREPARATION TIME: 5'   **COOKING TIME:** 0'   **SERVINGS:** 1

½ cup coconut milk
1 ½ cup water
½ Avocado fruit
2 packets Stevia, or as needed
1 cup Spring mix greens
1 Tbsp. avocado oil

1. Add all ingredients to a blender.
2. Blend until smooth and creamy.
3. Serve and enjoy.

NUTRITION: Calories 270, Fat 18, Fiber 1, Carbs 3, Protein 22

THE BERRY-LICIOUS AND HAZELNUT SMOOTHIE

PREPARATION TIME: 5'   COOKING TIME: 0'   SERVINGS: 1

1 tablespoon MCT oil
2 cup cold water
3 large blackberries, whole
1–2 packets Stevia, optional
2 Tbsp. chocolate powder, unsweetened
3 Tbsp. Hazelnut, chopped
1 Tbsp. heavy cream

1. Add all the listed ingredients to a blender.
2. Blend on high until smooth and creamy.
3. Enjoy your smoothie.

NUTRITION: Calories 350, Fat 8, Fiber 2, Carbs 8, Protein 26

PUMPKIN PIE BUTTERED COFFEE

PREPARATION TIME: 5'   COOKING TIME: 0'   SERVINGS: 1

12 oz. hot coffee
2 Tbsp. canned pumpkin
1 Tbsp. regular butter, unsalted
¼ tsp. pumpkin pie spice
Liquid stevia, to sweeten

1. Add listed ingredients to a blender
2. Blend until you have a smooth and creamy texture
3. Serve chilled and enjoy!

NUTRITION: Calories 200, Fat 8, Fiber 2, Carbs 8, Protein 36

THE BRAZILIAN NUTS SHAKE

PREPARATION TIME: 5'   **COOKING TIME:** 0'   **SERVINGS:** 1

1 Tbsp. sunflower seeds
1 cup water
1 oz. Brazil nuts
1 Tbsp. stevia
1 Tbsp. MCT oil
1 cup Spring mix salad blend

1. Add listed ingredients to a blender
2. Blend until you have a smooth and creamy texture
3. Serve chilled and enjoy!

NUTRITION: Calories 250, Fat 8, Fiber 2, Carbs 8, Protein 17

KETO FLU COMBAT SMOOTHIE

PREPARATION TIME: 5'   **COOKING TIME:** 15'   **SERVINGS:** 1

½ cup unsweetened nut or seed milk (hemp, almond, coconut, and cashew)
1 cup spinach
½ medium avocado (about 75 grams), pitted and peeled
1 scoop MCT powder (or 1 tablespoon MCT oil)
½ Tbsp. unsweetened cacao powder
¼ tsp. sea salt
Dash sweetener (optional)
½ cup ice

1. In a blender, combine the milk, spinach, avocado, MCT powder, cacao powder, salt, sweetener (if using), and ice, and blend until smooth.

NUTRITION: Calories 185, Fat 12, Fiber 2, Carbs 4, Protein 11

CHAPTER 14
Dessert Recipes

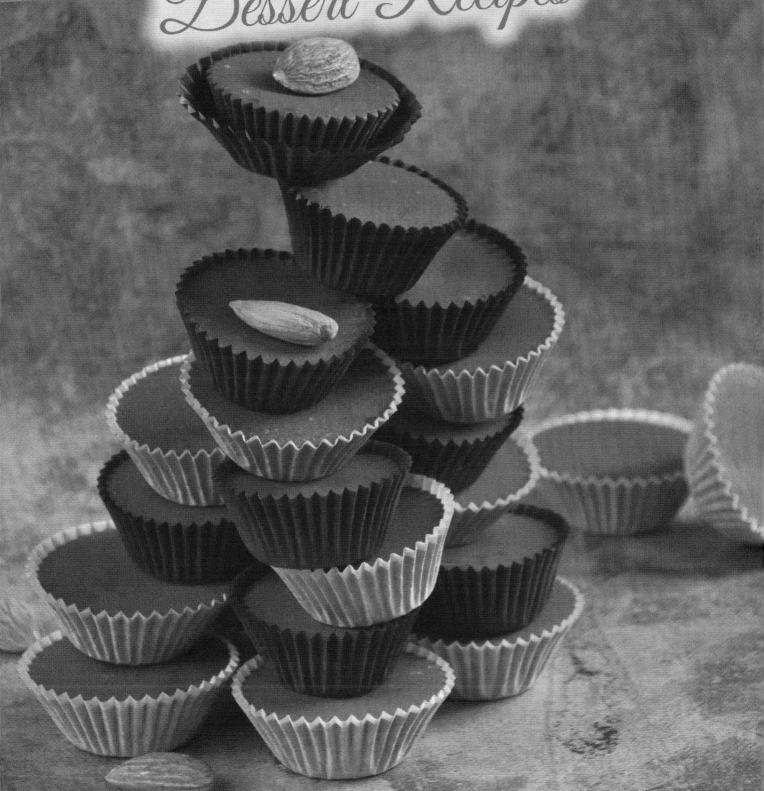

CHIA AND BLACKBERRY PUDDING

PREPARATION TIME: 6'   COOKING TIME: 30'   SERVINGS: 5

1 cup full-fat natural yogurt
2 tsp. swerve
2 Tbsp. chia seeds
1 cup fresh blackberries
1 Tbsp. lemon zest
Mint leaves, to serve

1. Mix together the yogurt and the swerve. Stir in the chia seeds. Reserve 4 blackberries for garnish and mash the remaining ones with a fork until pureed. Stir in the yogurt mixture
2. Chill in the fridge for 30 minutes.
3. When cooled, divide the mixture between 2 glasses.
4. Top each with a couple of blackberries, mint leaves, lemon zest, and serve.

NUTRITION: Calories 260, Fat 8, Fiber 2, Carbs 8, Protein 45

MINT CHOCOLATE PROTEIN SHAKE

PREPARATION TIME: 6'   COOKING TIME: 50'   SERVINGS: 5

3 cup flax milk, chilled
3 tsp. unsweetened cocoa powder
1 avocado, pitted, peeled, sliced
1 cup coconut milk, chilled
3 mint leaves + extra to garnish
3 Tbsp. erythritol
1 Tbsp. low carb Protein powder
Whipping cream, for topping

1. Combine the milk, cocoa powder, avocado, coconut milk, mint leaves, erythritol, and protein powder into a blender, and blend for 1 minute until smooth.
2. Pour into serving glasses, lightly add some whipping cream on top, and garnish with mint leaves.

NUTRITION: Calories 340, Fat 1, Fiber 2, Carbs 8, Protein 22

BOK CHOY MUSHROOM SOUP

PREPARATION TIME: 10'   **COOKING TIME:** 10'   **SERVINGS:** 10'

1 Chopped onion
Salt
2 Chopped celery stalk
6 cup Chicken stock
3 Tbsps. Coconut oil
2 bunches Quartered radishes
Black pepper
6 Minced garlic cloves

1. Set the pan over medium heat and preheat the oil
2. Stir in the celery, onion, and garlic to cook until soft, about 5 minutes
3. Stir in the stock, radishes, and seasonings.
4. Cover and simmer to boil for 15 minutes
5. Enjoy while still hot

NUTRITION: Calories: 131, Fat: 12, Fiber: 8, Carbs: 4, Protein: 1

ALMOND BUTTER FAT BOMBS

PREPARATION TIME: 6'   **COOKING TIME:** 30'   **SERVINGS:** 5

½ cup almond butter
½ cup coconut oil
4 Tbsp. unsweetened cocoa powder
½ cup erythritol

1. Melt butter and coconut oil in the microwave for 45 seconds, stirring twice until properly melted and mixed. Mix in cocoa powder and erythritol until completely combined.
2. Pour into muffin molds and refrigerate for 3 hours to harden.

NUTRITION: Calories 340, Fat 1, Fiber 2, Carbs 8, Protein 22

KETO PEANUT BUTTER CUP STYLE FUDGE

PREPARATION TIME: 10'   **COOKING TIME: 30'**   **SERVINGS: 36**

1 ½ cup natural peanut butter
¼ cup butter
¾ cup powdered swerve sweetener
1 tsp. vanilla extract
1/8 tsp. salt omit if butter is salted
3 Tbsp. peanuts chopped
Flaked sea salt, for topping

1. Line a baking sheet with parchment pepper for easy removal.
2. Add peanut butter, vanilla, and butter to a pan, and heat over medium heat until melted and smooth.
3. Turn off the heat and stir in sweetener and salt, combine to mix well.
4. Spread the mixture in the prepared baking sheet in an even layer.
5. Chill for 20–30 minutes, cut into 36 slices.
6. Sprinkle with sea salt or other toppings of your choice, keep in an airtight container.

NUTRITION: Calories 100, Fat 7, Fiber 2, Carbs 8, Protein 6

CHOCOLATE MACADAMIA NUT FAT BOMBS

PREPARATION TIME: 11'   **COOKING TIME: 30'**   **SERVINGS: 4**

1 1/3 oz. (38g) sugar-free dark chocolate
1 Tbsp. coconut oil
Coarse salt or sea salt
1 ½ oz. (42 g.) raw macadamia nuts halves

1. Put 3 macadamia nut halves in each of 8 wells of the mini muffin pan.
2. Microwave the chocolate chips for about a few seconds.
3. Whisk until smooth, add coconut oil and salt, mix until well combined.
4. Fill the mini muffin pan with the chocolate mixture to cover the nuts completely.
5. Refrigerate the muffin pan until chilled and firm, for about 30 minutes.

NUTRITION: Calories 100, Fat 7, Fiber 2, Carbs 8, Protein 6

KETO PEANUT BUTTER CHOCOLATE BARS

PREPARATION TIME: **11'**   COOKING TIME: **10'**   SERVINGS: **8**

For the bars:
¾ cup (84 g.) superfine almond flour
2 oz. (56.7 g.) butter
¼ cup (45.5 g.) swerve, icing sugar style
½ cup peanut butter
1 tsp. vanilla extract

For the topping:
½ cup (90 g.) sugar-free chocolate chips

1. Combine all the ingredients for the bars and spread them into a small 6-inch pan.
2. Microwave the chocolate in the microwave oven for 30 seconds and whisk until smooth.
3. Pour the melted chocolate over the bars' ingredients.
4. Refrigerate for at least an hour or 2 until the bars firmed. Keep in an airtight container.

NUTRITION: Calories 200, Fat 8, Fiber 2, Carbs 8, Protein 6

CHAPTER 15
Keto Diet Success Stories

SUSAN ANDREW – 50 YEARS

My name is Susan and at 50 years old, I can still clearly picture the very first time I was teased and bullied in school about my weight. I was in the seventh grade. I had always been a chubby kid growing up. In my family, everyone was chubby and so, until that moment, it had never been a source of shame for me. A new kid, to fit in, had started picking on me to gain popularity, and this had started a new trend for myself. I completely isolated myself from that moment and was always alone. I avoided at all costs being around my schoolmates when I ate because they would tease me so much.

When I could not find a safe spot at school to hide and have my lunch, I stopped eating at school altogether. This resulted in me getting home later on and going on a binge eating all that I came across until when I went to bed. This went on for years and by the time I was graduating high school, I was already overweight. I went to college and my feelings of rejection which had caused me to isolate myself only became worse. I hid out in my room only coming out for classes and never participating in any way socially. I was always in constant fear that if I let myself I would be ridiculed and bullied, and therefore, I kept it to myself as much as possible.

With the added isolation came more and more weight gain and when finally graduated college, I weighed 345lbs. This went on to when I got married and had a family. My wake-up call came in form of a sharp pain which rendered me motionless at the age of 30. I ended up in a hospital and I was diagnosed with rheumatoid arthritis. I suddenly was in severe pain and could not even hold my child. I knew it was time to let go of the past and make some changes. I took it upon myself to seek both healing in my body and my mind. I knew deep down one of the reasons why I never tried losing weight in earnest before was because a part of me was still stuck in those years when I was teased as a child because of being overweight. I sought professional help and for three days and a week, I saw my doctor religiously to sort out my fears and heal from my past.

I then went to work on researching the best ways to lose weight because I wanted a method that I could do with my family and not affect their lifestyle too much. It was an old friend I had reconnected with as part of my healing journey who encouraged me to try out the Ketogenic diet. I had done it also and it had helped me lose a good amount of weight just in time for my wedding and I told everyone who could listen how great the ketogenic diet was.

After doing my research, I felt comfortable choosing the diet. This was ideal because I could eat and did not have to skip any meals because my life was demanding and I needed my energy levels to be high during the day. I began by changing my eating habits from greasy high-calorie fast foods and junk foods to more healthy balanced meals we could enjoy as a family. I cleared all the snacks that were unhealthy and began packing small tubs of healthy vegetable smacks to have whenever I felt the cravings coming in.

I did not completely stop indulging in my beloved fast food but only limited it to once a week. This helped me not to go on a binge. The first time I started the Ketogenic diet, on a particularly challenging day, I had fallen off the wagon and binged on a lot of junk food. I researched and learned it was common because I was feeling very guilty. I saw a lot of people talking about having one or two cheat meals per week so that you do not fall back to old habits. This worked and soon I found myself going for two weeks without indulging in junk foods.

I had started out weighing 371lbs and had dropped the 71lbs in 10 months after being dedicated to the Ketogenic diet. My rheumatoid arthritis eased as the weight came off and I was full of energy. My counseling sessions also played a big role in boosting my self-esteem by letting go of the past. I continued with my ketogenic diet journey till now to reach my goal which is 225lbs.

EMILY WILLIAMS - 52 YEARS

I had worn the same huge clothes for more than ten years. I never had the heart to go out shopping because nothing would fit me anyway. No matter how much my daughter Christine tried to encourage me to go shopping, I always came up with an excuse. I was always tired and out of breath and did as little as possible which meant spending less time with my vibrant daughter who would soon be leaving for college.

It wasn't always like this. Yes, I had been big most of my adult life, but not obese to the extent that it hurt me at times to simply walk. At work, I was always at my desk and tried to move as little as possible and even though my boss was a gracious man, I knew my weight and the related complications were hindering my performance. Most of the people I had started with at the company had been promoted and even moved to better positions, but I was still where I had started. It was simply depressing for me.

1 had started eating more after my husband had passed away, leaving me with two children to fend for. I had moved closer to his place of work and my own family lived far away. This had plunged me into a state of loneliness when became a widow. I had slowly started using food as my escape from all the stress and pressure of being a full-time working single mum. The weight kept piling on and on, and now I was at a point where I did not know what to do anymore. I desired to spend more time with my daughter before leaving for college.

This is what inspired me to find out how to lose weight once and for all. I had to admit to myself that all my previous attempts at different diets and exercise plans were halfhearted attempts. I never stuck to any of them for more than a week and always found myself plunged back to old harmful habits. Now, my kids were all grown up and my first was about to leave. Would I even be able to go and visit her in college if I kept my lifestyle the same? The truth was I couldn't.

My doctor was also another reason for realizing I had to make changes in my life. He was concerned about my very high cholesterol levels which were affecting my heart. If things did not change, the future looked bleak, to say the least. I knew I had some reflection to do and finally, I had to find a way to not only lose the weight but be able to keep it off as well. It was my daughter Christine who introduced me to the Ketogenic diet. The mum of a friend had lost a good amount of weight with it, and it was easier to do than most of my diets and fads. They began researching on it and I got started.

Getting myself to commit to it for one month was going to be an uphill task. I was a constant procrastinator and never saw many projects through. I needed to come up with enough strength to give the ketogenic diet my all and, therefore, I made spending more quality time with my vibrant children my driving force. I admitted I had completely given up on myself. That is why I never even tried dating again because I just did not want to try. Even my own children at some point encouraged me to get back to myself and date again but always had excuses on why I couldn't. Now that they were both about to leave, be it two years apart, I had run out of excuses and soon would be alone. This meant a new chapter in my life and I wanted deep down for it to be a great chapter and no longer depressing.

One of the first changes we made was to change our diet as a family. My children were not plus size but they wanted to support me and therefore they joined me in cleaning up what they all ate. There were no more greasy foods allowed in the house, which meant no more ordering food. They had to cook at home. I began also being more active with walking more on my way from and to work which was not too far from where I lived. I found that with the Ketogenic diet, my mind had more clarity and I was actually being more focused at work as well.

The greatest benefit as the weight began to drop was being able to participate in the activities my children were interested in. The first time I went to the mall with my daughter and tried on a dress and it actually fit and made me completely break down. This meant I was on the right track. My doctor was very happy with the results of my falling cholesterol levels as well. I began reconnecting with old friends who, I must admit, I was always hiding from whenever they came to invite me to the community events that were held every now and then.

As my daughter was leaving for college, I had been on the ketogenic diet for 6 months and had lost a total of 63lbs which was a tremendous amount. I was able to drive her to school and get her settled. We enjoyed our time together because I no longer felt exhausted all day long and had more energy to keep up. I still have a long way to go aiming at losing 100lbs but I know now that I can do it, I'm more outgoing and social now more than I have ever been in a long time.

JANE HILL – 54 YEARS

Thanks to the Ketogenic diet, I had moved from a size 28 to a size 13. This did not happen overnight but it took me 2 long years full of all the challenges, both physical and mental, imaginable. I had dedicated my life obsessively to the ketogenic diet and for the first year, it was all I could do. I was unable to exercise due to complications with an old injury from high school which had gotten worse the bigger I had become over the years.

When graduated from college, I was overweight due to all the bad habits involved in my adventures while traveling and my love for takeout as well. I had finally fallen into the obese category when the stresses of the outside world had finally caught up with me. I was no longer a carefree college girl, but now had bills to pay and a stressful demanding job in a top law firm. I had to work strenuous hours and simply had no time to care for myself at all. The constant traveling did not help me because it reduced my chances of getting a healthy meal and I devolved more into junk foods and eating out.

It was when I was traveling for work and had a health scare that I realized I needed to make some changes in my life. Being in a foreign country and unwell so far from all that was safe and familiar was very scary. My doctor was a no-nonsense gentleman who came in and told my point-blank that I either lose weight or simply changed careers to something more comfortable at home. With an increase in my weight and the added stress, I was not going to like where my health ended up in a couple of years. He suggested I take some time off to distress and decide on what to do. When I flew back home, I did just that and took my leave.

I reflected and knew that even though my job was demanding and very stressful, I actually enjoyed it and wanted to keep traveling as well. Then, it was my weight that needed to go. While traveling in one of the airport lounges, I had happened upon an article in one of the magazines talking about the ketogenic diet and a lady was telling her story of how had lost tremendous amounts of weight. I had been uninterested at the time but now I started doing more research on it in earnest.

I learned more about ketogenic which has been around for centuries. I wanted to do it right and learn as much as I could before getting back to work. I learned all the information available about the benefits of fasting and basically consumed all success stories could find on people who had used ketogenic to lose weight. I even found people who had demanding lives like mine and noted down all the tricks they used to keep on track as they went about their full days. I learned also about all the health risks associated with being obese and made more effort to visit my doctor who seconded that I truly needed to do something to shed weight to keep myself healthy.

My research was based a lot on calorie reduction. I learned how to count the number of calories in the foods taken which were important to losing weight. It was possible to add weight even while doing the ketogenic diet if you did not reduce the number of calories you consumed. I would pick a day, especially on Sunday, when I was at home, and prepare meals for the coming week in advance. This ensured I chose the right ingredients and prepared the meals to be very healthy. When I would come home from work too exhausted to cook which earlier meant calling for takeout, now I had prepared a meal which all I needed to do was warm and eat.

It was when I was traveling that I was most challenged. I researched healthy snack options that I carried with me and got to know all the healthy meal options in advance at where I was staying. This was a lot of work but I was determined to get to my goal, and so I kept going. My doctor one day told me I had moved on from being obese to being overweight and for someone who had chosen to avoid the scale, I felt I was on the right path. 2 years later, I weighed less than I ever had and was a beautiful size 14. I actually began a chat group at work to support my colleagues not only in my home company but in all their branches. They had come to me when they saw my amazing transformation. Their interest has kept me going and helped me learn more about weight loss and living a healthier journey in the long run. I learned that once you lose weight, it is important to keep yourself accountable, otherwise, you can easily revert to old habits.

CONCLUSION

The ketogenic diet is a diet that believes that by minimizing your carbs while maximizing the good fat in your system and making sure that you're getting the protein you need, you will be happier and healthier. In this book, we give you the information to know what this diet is all about, as well as describing the different types and areas that this diet will offer. Most people assume that there is only one way to do this and while there is one thing that the additional options share, there are actually four different options you can choose from. Each one has its unique benefits, and you should know about each type to learn what would be best for your body, which is why we have described them in the book for you to have the best information possible when you begin this diet for yourself.

If you are faced with any difficult situations when following the keto diet, you should remind yourself of why you started the keto diet, to begin with, and what you are hoping to see from your diet health-wise or lifestyle-wise. No matter what your reason is for starting the keto diet, you should focus on that and try to put difficult situations behind you. If you are still having trouble coping with a certain situation, then you can always ask for advice from one of your keto groups or your like-minded friends. You never know, they might have some great advices for you.

The next step is to begin your keto journey and start your new life. Women over 50 need to take better care of themselves than ever before; so, if you have not made yourself your top priority before, please do so now. Now is the time for you to adopt the keto lifestyle and do everything in your power to make yourself better physically and mentally. Get your diet in order, begin an exercise routine, and start caring for you, the most crucial person in your life.

This book has given you all the information you need to do this diet properly and to do it well. It's important to understand what you're getting into when you go into this diet, and this book will give you valuable information that you can use to your benefit, and so you can avoid the problems that can come with this diet. You want to stay healthy and make sure that your body can do what it needs to. As with anything, we have put a strong emphasis on the fact that if anything feels wrong or unnatural you will need to see a doctor to make sure that you are safe and that your body can handle this diet. Use the knowledge in this book to have amazing recipes and learn how to prepare amazing meals for yourself.